TO ALIGHTA

A VOTRE SANTÉ

How to Lower Your Cholesterol With French Gourmet Food

A practical guide

By Chef Alain Braux

C.E.P.C., C.M.B.

B.S. Holistic Nutrition

Business Page

"The only packaged food I believe in is whole foods coming in Nature's own packaging." -*Mike Adams, NaturalNews.com*

Copyright © 2009 by Alain Braux International Publishing, LLC.

All rights reserved. No part of this book may be reproduced or transmitted in any forms or by any means, electronic or mechanical, including photocopying, recording or by any form of information storage and retrieval system, without the written permission of the author except where permitted by law.

EAN-13: 9781448676972

ISBN-10: 1448676975

How to Lower your Cholesterol with French Gourmet Food is a trademark of Alain Braux, Alain Braux International Publishing, LLC.

Disclaimer: This publication contains the opinions and ideas of its author. It is intended to provide helpful and informative material regarding the subject addressed in this guide. It is sold with the understanding that the author and publisher are not engaged in rendering medical, health, psychological, or any other kind of personal professional services in this guide. If you, the reader, require personal medical, health, or other professional assistance or advice, you are advised to consult your physician or other qualified professional.

The author and publisher specifically disclaim all responsibility for any liability, loss, or risk, personal or otherwise, that is incurred as a consequence, directly or indirectly, of the use and application of any of the contents of this guide.

Before starting a new diet plan or lifestyle change, or beginning or modifying an exercise program, please check with your personal physician to make sure that the changes you plan to make are right for you. Sincerely, Alain Braux.

For information regarding this and other Alain Braux International Publishing, LLC books and speaking engagements, please contact Alain Braux through AlainBraux.com or alainbraux@gmail.com

Cover design by **Nathan Stueve**.

Front and back photographs by **Athena Danoy**.

Manufactured in the United States of America. (August 2009)

TABLE OF CONTENTS

FOREWORD

I first met Alain Braux in 2002 when he came to cook for our family. Alain is an extraordinary chef who serves superb food that is healthy and pleasing to all the senses.

Alain has seen healthy food work magic in his own life. He has a passionate commitment to make healthy food taste delicious. Years ago when the Pritikin diet was popular for lowering cholesterol everybody who tried it would complain, "Yuck, like straw, tasteless." One won't find that to be true of Alain's recipes. It's more like, "Delicious! Is this really healthy for me?"

"How to Lower your Cholesterol with French Gourmet Food. A Practical Guide" delivers a perspective on food that is exciting and practical. Alain begins with his own experience and before you know it you are in the pantry wanting to duplicate his recipes. The reader is taken on a health journey through the world of good food and receives Alain's firsthand account of his challenge to improve his own health through diet.

This book is an excellent resource for anybody trying to improve their health with a goal of enhancing their digestion, decreasing their waistline and improving their fat metabolism. Alain has a sharp eye for all things delicious and a command of healthy cooking techniques that are unparalleled.

English is Alain's second language. That he wrote this book in his second language is a testimonial to his passion to communicate his unique and effective ideas. I am grateful to Alain for creating this for people all over the world who want to eat delicious food, lower their cholesterol and achieve vital health.

In good health,

Janet Zand, L.Ac., OMD, Dipl. Ac., Dipl. CH, ACN

How Can This Book Help You?

Who Is Alain Braux?

Bonjour. My name is Alain Braux and I am a classically trained French chef and a formally educated Nutritherapist. Two years ago I was diagnosed with high cholesterol, and I managed to bring my cholesterol levels down by returning to the food ways of my youth in Southern France. I lowered my cholesterol significantly with diet alone, and I wrote this book to let you know how you can do it, too.

You might wonder: what's a nice Frenchman like me doing in Texas? Suffice it to say that I followed my chef's nose and sense of adventure from job to job, and together they brought me halfway across the globe. I have been working in the food business in different capacities for the past 40 years and loved all the different aspects of it.

I started my career by doing my apprenticeship in a Swiss Confiserie in Nice, France. Following that, I worked in assorted pastry shops, as well as four-star palaces on the Cote d'Azur such as **Le Grand Hotel du Cap d'Antibes** near Cannes and **l'Hôtel Negresco** in Nice. I also worked in several top restaurants such as **Le Moulin de Mougins** near Cannes, **Lenotre** in Paris, and two of finest pastry shops in Brussels, Belgium: **Espagne** and **Wittamer**.

I then crossed the pond to come to America. In New York City, I worked at the **Dumas Pastry Shop** and **Délices La Cote Basque**, then moved down to Houston to help open and operate the American **Lenotre**, a branch of the famous Parisian patisserie. I came to Austin to work with Judy Willcott at **Texas French Bread**, and eventually opened my own shop: **Amandine French Bakery and Café**. After I lost my business (alas, a good chef does not necessarily make a good businessman), I became the Executive Pastry Chef at **Barr Mansion**, and taught Pastry and Baking Arts at the **Culinary Academy of Austin**. I finally landed as the Executive Chef and Nutritherapist at **People's Pharmacy**, where I currently create and produce healthy food, including desserts, for customers with food allergies. I also have a nutrition consulting business called **A Votre Santé** (To Your Health), where I design menus and dietary guidelines for clients with food sensitivities. I also teach gluten and dairy-free baking classes at **Whole Foods Market** and **Central Market** in Austin.

My Nutritional Background

About 10 years ago, when I was running my own business, I became interested in nutrition, thanks to a couple of vegetarian assistants. They were commenting on the fact that I was not offering vegetarian dishes at my lunch counter. In Austin, a lot of people are health conscious, as well as thoughtful about their food choices. As a French-trained chef, my only concern was to offer the best tasting product. I was not trained in the arcane of nutrition. But as I devised increasingly health-conscious dishes, I became more intrigued by the effect on food on one's health. After I had to close my business and began searching for a new direction in life, I started to think: wouldn't it be great if I could combine my 30 years of knowledge as a chef and my newfound interest in nutrition?

Right around that time I heard an advertisement on the radio for a new Macrobiotic school: **The Natural Epicurean Academy**. I enrolled, and after studying there for two years, I became a Macrobiotic and Natural Food Specialist. As fascinating and enlightening as it was, I found this particular Japanese-based diet philosophy a little limiting. I decided to widen my nutrition horizon by studying for a B.S. of Holistic Nutrition at the **Clayton College of Holistic Health**.

What Is A Nutritherapist?

I prefer to use the European designation to differentiate myself from Nutritionists. You see, the vast majority of nutritionists work exclusively with vitamins and supplements. While supplements are a good way to help you improve your health, prescribing pills is not what I do with my private clientele. A nutritherapist, on the other hand, works exclusively with *food and food only* to help his/her clients with their health conditions. I believe firmly that the vast majority of our modern degenerative diseases are self-generated, and result from the effects of bad basic nutrition. Whether we are eating too much fast food or commercially prepared foods, drinking overly sweet soft drinks or stuffing ourselves with snacks loaded with trans-fatty acids and high fructose corn syrup, we are harming ourselves through our daily food choices.

There are many reasons for this: lack of basic nutrition education in school; our government's lack of focus on the prevention of disease; the constant barrage of marketing brainwashing we are subjected to since childhood; the fact that this society is constantly on the run and busy, busy, busy. We do not take the time to prepare a good and healthy meal. We do not take the time to enjoy that meal with our family or friends. We are way too rushed to pay attention to the essential things in our lives: food and love. Our jobs and assorted obligations force us to be constantly on the run and harried. Ours is a busy and productive, but not a healthy society.

My Goal For You

My goal is to provide the information and education you need to understand what cholesterol is, and how it affects you; to tell you about an assortment of foods that will help you live more healthfully and lower your cholesterol; to explain how and where to shop for these foods; to provide you with a health plan based on the foods that can help lower your cholesterol; and, finally, to provide you with an assortment of Mediterranean and French recipes not only good for your health, but also full of flavor. My wish for you is that this book will help you in your goal to live a happy and healthy life without the need for a cocktail of chemical healing. A Votre Santé (To Your Health) and Bonne Chance (good luck) with this program!

What This Book Is

I have designed this book as a practical guide. It is a nutrition/cookbook hybrid. It contains a great deal of nutrition information specifically targeted on lowering serum cholesterol and recipes to help you apply this information. As a chef and nutritherapist, my wish is to provide practical information you can use in your daily life. I will try not to overwhelm you with scientific information, just giving you enough to let you know why I make my recommendations. If you wish to dig deeper into the nutritional details of each food, there is plenty of information out there for you to consult. I will also include some of my personal reasons why I chose these foods, as well as offer you Chef's tricks, shortcuts and anecdotes. I picked some of my favorite recipes for your culinary enjoyment. I also tried to keep them short and easy to prepare. But please remember that, in the long run, our health is the most important asset we have. Without it, there is not a whole lot we can do. We won't be able to work and we lose income. We won't be able to fully enjoy life, our family and friends. Not to mention all the money we end up paying to doctors, hospitals and health insurance. Keeping your body healthy should be your major focus, not an afterthought. Daily food maintenance is the key to your good health.

My Food Beliefs

I read this quote once and it absolutely describes how I feel: "The only packaged food I believe in is whole foods coming in Nature's own packaging." -Mike Adams, NaturalNews.com.

One of my heroes, Dr. Seignalet, the famous French immunologist, called his masterpiece work "Alimentation ou la Troisième Médecine" or "Food or the Third Medicine". Although I absolutely agree with his vision that food can be one of the ways to heal ourselves - the other two modern ways of healing being allopathic Western medicine and alternative medicine - I firmly believe that being healthy and staying that way should be accomplished through food FIRST.

For too long, we have been trained to believe that the only way to stay healthy is to trust the modern medicine way of healing through chemical medication and physical surgery. I believe that it is the wrong way to look at it. If we feed our body's healthy food to begin with, we are less likely to need these harsh treatments.

I do agree that modern medicine can be useful in cases of emergency. If you break your arm, going to the emergency room is the best way to treat that broken bone. But you should help the healing along with good quality food. I also agree that, in some cases, supplementation is necessary to remedy a lack of a specific vitamin or mineral. Such a lack, however, often points to an imbalance in your basic diet. Ideally - and I do know we don't live in an ideal world - we should get all of our nutrients from our food.

In our modern society, our feeding habits have been so influenced by the constant marketing of what they call "food" that we don't know how to eat an everyday, balanced diet anymore. Our fast-paced lifestyle forces us to eat on the run, swallow fast food and reheat convenience industrialized meals loaded with chemical and artificial flavorings, colorings and preservatives. Let's be honest about it: many commercially-prepared foods are woefully low in nutrients. Heating these foods in microwave ovens can further reduce what little nutritional value they began with. We are eating nutritionally-dead food and we wonder why we are hungry two hours after eating a meal? Our body wants and needs real and nutritious food to function. With such a meal, we have filled our bodies with empty calories and all sorts of chemical junk. Of course it wants more! Then, because we feel a lack of energy, we eat a sweetened snack to keep us going until the next empty meal and so on, and so forth. After a few years of abuse, our body starts to break down and degenerative diseases are starting to show up: heartburn, digestive problems, hypoglycemia, type 2 diabetes, weight gain, high cholesterol, high blood pressure, heart problems, strokes and cancer, to name a few. Of course! What do we expect? We feed our body junk and as wonderful a living machine as it was created, it starts breaking down due to the abuse we subject it to. Most of you know that if you fill your car with regular gasoline when it's supposed to run on premium, eventually your engine will start to malfunction, gunk up and eventually break down. It amazes me that the vast majority of people in this country maintain their bodies more poorly than their cars. And they wonder why they get sick!

What we need is to slow down, pay attention to our body's basic needs, and take good care of it as we would our car and fuel it properly. Our body is our temple and as such, we should show it utmost respect, love and care. Please love your body the way it deserves and it will take care of itself. The result will be a good and long lasting health.

From a purely economic point of view, eating healthy to stay healthy also makes perfect sense. As I have told my son repeatedly, I prefer to spend a little more money now while enjoying good-tasting healthy food than spend all my money later in expensive supplements, health insurance premiums, doctor's treatments or hospital bills. Why not enjoy life and the good health provided to us by nature, and prevent disease in the process? Being sick is not our natural state. Given the opportunity and good quality food, our immune system will keep us strong and healthy for a long time. Unfortunately, our society has taught us to think short term and not in terms of prevention and long-term health.

Take Back Your Power of Self-care

I believe that we should all regain control of our own health through self-care. We must take back what is ours - our power to decide what is in the best interest of our health. Yes, we need professional guidance to help us make these decisions, but the final decision should be ours. For too long, we have abdicated our health decisions to others. It is time to take that power back and be responsible for our own health choices. We need to take responsibility for how we treat and feed our bodies.

Health Coverage In America

It is not a secret that the health care costs in this country are outrageous. If you're lucky, you are covered by your company's group health insurance. Even if you can afford to pay the premium, you end up paying good money for assorted deductibles and procedures that are not covered by your plan. And that is, if you have health insurance. It is a well-known fact that millions of people in this country – the most advanced country in the world – either are not offered insurance coverage by their company because it's too expensive or, if they are out of work, cannot afford to pay for any form of health insurance. Although I'm fully aware that I'm simplifying things here, wouldn't it make sense to take the best care we can of ourselves, to at least keep the costs down?

Health Starts In The Gut; Or, That Gut Feeling

In our modern days, it seems the wisdom of the gut is lost. For centuries, it has been known that health begins and ends in the gut. Many of our modern degenerative diseases start with a damaged digestive system. How we treat our stomach, our small intestine, and our colon determines how we ultimately feel overall. Modern medicine focuses too much on the symptoms of after-the-fact health issues; I believe we need to start thinking about proper digestive system maintenance first. What's the use of "fixing" an unlimited list of symptoms after the fact, if we do not pay attention to the basics first? Heal the gut and the symptoms will eventually disappear. Acid reflux, heartburn and GERD are due to your stomach's ill health. Many digestive problems can be traced back to damage caused to our small intestine. Illnesses such as IBS (irritable bowel syndrome), Crohn's disease and colon cancer have been linked to the type of foods we ingest. Treat your gut well, and it will return the favor.

How We Eat, Not Just What We Eat, Is Important To Digestive Health

In our stressed-out, fast-fast-fast society where we feel that the more we do and the faster we do it is a good thing; the speed of our lives is one of the ways we make ourselves sick. Eating on the run, eating while standing up (sur le pouce in French) or worse, eating "fast" food while driving (by the way, is it fast because it's prepared quickly, or because we scarf down that "food" in less than 5 minutes?) while we rush from one appointment to another across town.

Old-fashioned wisdom has it right. Take your time to eat and enjoy your food. There are many reasons for this: first, our food should be chewed properly, so that we puree our food in very small pieces. Remember, your stomach does not have teeth; it cannot do this for you. Another reason for thorough chewing is it allows our salivary enzymes, salivary amylase and ptyalin, to start the digestive process, especially of carbohydrates. The macrobiotic philosophy suggests that we chew each bite of food at least 50 times before we swallow it. I know who has the time? But we should still make an effort.

Another thing to be avoided is eating under stress. Taking a 30-minute lunch break is too short to allow us to eat our food calmly and with awareness; an hour is better. Better yet, in the South of France - before the advent of air conditioning - we used to stop working from noon to 3 pm to allow us to go back home, eat a homemade meal in a leisurely manner with our families and even take a nap after that. It's still done this way in small villages where traffic doesn't prevent you from going home for lunch. When I was an apprentice in 1969, I heard a Parisian couple complaining about us lazy Southerners because we were taking a 3-hour lunch break and the store was closed. In the minds of big city folks, this was unacceptable. Having been through the 8-hour (and longer) shifts in this country, I now realize the wisdom of our Southern tradition. We first start by whetting the appetite with an aperitif - if you're old enough - or une menthe a l'eau (mint-flavored water) if you're young. While we wait for the food to be ready, we have a nice conversation. We then enjoy a light meal accompanied with a lively discussion, a nice strong (but small) espresso coffee and even, on special days, a pousse-café (after-coffee digestive liquor). Now that's living!

When eating, there should be no distraction from the enjoyment of food but good company. No TV, no computer, no reading books or magazines. We should focus on chewing our food.

My Own Cholesterol Story

This book began with the idea of sharing my personal cholesterol-lowering experience. A few years ago, I accepted a position as a pastry and baking instructor at a culinary school. It sounded like a perfect fit for me; after all, I had been a pastry chef for more than 30 years at the time. What I did not realize was that this was a whole new career. I had never been a teacher before, nor had I ever trained to be one. I had to learn, very quickly, to create curriculums, write lesson plans, speak in public and actually explain how things are done in a professional kitchen. It was a new and very stressful situation. Stress is a known factor in increasing cholesterol levels.

To make things worse, I had to grade my students on the quality of their work. That meant having to taste pastries and baked goods more or less every day. I know what you're thinking: What a job! Who wouldn't want to eat sweet desserts every day? In the beginning, it was fun, but then I noticed that my body started to resist tasting pastries. The taste and even the idea of eating sugar made me gag. A normal reaction to any overdose, whether an illegal drug or sugar. In fact, some people believe that sugar is a powerfully addictive product. What I didn't know was that, unbeknownst to me, my cholesterol level was going higher and higher. Excess sugar can produce a significant rise in triglycerides, promote an elevation of low-density lipoproteins (LDL, the so called "bad" cholesterol) and reduce high density lipoproteins (HDL, the "good" cholesterol).

On top of that, my daily diet was erratic. To deal with the fatigue and stress of a new job, I got into the habit of drinking too much coffee - the mountain-grown type - brewed in (what else?) a French press, of course. I learned much later through personal research that coffee brewed as espresso, Turkish-style or French-style, although very flavorful, contains a compound called cafestol. Cafestol is known to elevate LDL cholesterol and triglyceride levels. It appears that using paper coffee filters take most of the cafestol out.

To add insult to injury, because I was working hard to learn my new trade, I made a habit of working through lunch, eating canned soup directly from the can. As you can imagine, these bad habits did not help my health. I started having terrible heartburn and, to my dismay, at my annual check-up, I discovered that my cholesterol level had shot up to 240. While it's not terribly high, it was still 40 points above what is considered to be "normal". What's more important, it was way higher than it had been. My job was damaging my health.

Through my side business as a Nutritherapist, I met my next boss, Bill Swail, the owner of **People's Pharmacy**. In addition to being a regular pharmacy, **People's** has a great reputation in Austin for its alternative healing programs, such as nutritional advice, chiropractic services, supplements and homeopathy. It also provides custom-designed pharmaceutical compounds and offers wholesome quality food.

It was a match made in heaven. Bill offered me a position as a chef and Nutritherapist. My responsibility is to create healthy dishes as well as custom-designed food and desserts for people with certain food allergies such as gluten and dairy. I also create low-sugar desserts for customers with hypoglycemia and diabetes. I am able to continue to consult privately with people needing special dietary assistance, as well.

How I Lowered My Cholesterol Levels

When I began my new job at **People's Pharmacy**, I decided to mend my ways and return to the healthy road I should never have left. Knowing my cholesterol had gotten too high, I resolved to use myself as a guinea pig and lower my cholesterol through diet and lifestyle improvements alone. I went back to what I knew best, the French Mediterranean home cooking of my youth… and it worked. As you can see from the chart below, I still have some work to do, but I made remarkable and significant improvement.

My Test Results Numbers

After a year of improving my diet and lifestyle, my numbers looked as follows:

	2007	2008	Results	Comments
Total Cholesterol	240	205	35 points drop	Good
LDL	167	143	24 points drop	Very Good
HDL	52	49	3 points drop	Not As Good
Triglycerides	105	67	38 points drop	Very Good
Ratio LDL/HDL	3.21:1	2.91:1	Lower is better	Very Good. Below 3:1 is best
Ratio Total Cholesterol /HDL	4.62:1	4.18:1	Lower is better	Very Good. Below 5:1 is best

My own short analysis is:

- Total Cholesterol: Good, but still some work to do. Continue to watch my diet.
- Triglycerides: Very good. A good drop, due to the fact that I stopped eating sweet pastries daily.
- LDL ("bad") Cholesterol: Very good. A good drop, but can be improved. Keep on going!
- HDL ("good") Cholesterol: Could have been better. It should have increased. I'll have to keep working on it.

- Total Cholesterol/HDL and LDL/HDL ratios: Both of them are very good. I like to look at these numbers, as they are a better indication of the whole picture.

Although the goal is to decrease your total cholesterol level, the more important goal is to decrease LDL, increase HDL and lower your ratios. And remember, I did all of this without the help of statins or any other drugs. The only changes I made were to my diet and my lifestyle.

What Is Cholesterol?

To understand what healthy cholesterol levels are, you must understand what cholesterol is. It is a modified fat that is actually more like wax than fat or oil; it does not dissolve readily in water or in your bloodstream. Between 1,500 and 1,800 mg (1.5 to 1.8 grams) of cholesterol are produced every day by your body. Most of it is manufactured by your liver and smaller amounts by your small intestine and body cells. Between 200 and 800 mg daily come from the Standard American Diet (SAD). If you eliminated all cholesterol from your diet, your body would increase its production. If this substance is so dangerous, why would your body produce it? Because it can't function without it!

Why Is It Important For Your Body?

It might surprise you to learn that cholesterol performs a lot of essential functions in your body. You need cholesterol to survive. Every cell uses cholesterol to help construct protective cell membranes. It helps cells maintain their shape, and at the same time forms a special barrier against various toxic substances, making cells resistant to the penetration of certain toxins and keeping water from leaving your body too quickly.

Cholesterol also provides the basis of several important steroid hormones produced in the adrenal glands, ovaries, and testes. It is also necessary to help produce vitamin D every time we take in some sun during the day.

Is Cholesterol Bad For You?

In and of itself, cholesterol is not the bad substance it has been made to seem so by the medical establishment. We could not survive without cholesterol. It is true that excess cholesterol coming from your diet may be unhealthy for you, but the real cause of health troubles is when this cholesterol is oxidized by free radicals. Then it can become dangerous. That is why eating foods rich in antioxidants is so important. Foods rich in antioxidants, such as those with vitamins E, C and beta carotene, can help prevent the oxidation of cholesterol and the damage it may cause to blood vessels.

Some scientists believe that damage caused by the numerous toxins we ingest and breathe daily is causing inflammations that damage our arteries. When the body notices these inflammations, it tries to fix the small tears created in our arteries by patching them up with cholesterol. Over the years, these accumulations of cholesterol are causing plaque and artery blockage, potentially causing atherosclerosis, heart attacks or strokes from lack of blood flow to our heart and brain.

How is Cholesterol Involved with Atherosclerosis?

Cholesterol can move in the bloodstream only by being transported by LDL. The LDL molecule has a globular shape with a hollow core. Its job is to carry cholesterol throughout our body where it's needed to generate brain tissues, vitamin D, and so on. At this point, cholesterol in the bloodstream is neither good nor bad. It's just cholesterol.

Atherosclerosis develops when these low-density lipoprotein molecules (LDL), also labeled "bad" cholesterol, become oxidized by oxygen free radicals contained in our arteries' blood. Since our arteries' job is to carry oxygen to our heart, this is where atherosclerosis tends to develop. Blood in veins contains little oxygen, so atherosclerosis rarely develops there. When oxidized LDL cholesterol comes in contact with an artery wall, a series of reactions occur.

Our body, trying to repair the damage to the artery wall caused by oxidized LDL, calls on your immune system for help. It sends an army of specialized white blood cells (macrophages and T-lymphocytes) to absorb the oxidized-

LDL, forming specialized foam cells. Unfortunately, these white blood cells are not able to process the oxidized-LDL, and ultimately grow then rupture, depositing a greater amount of oxidized cholesterol onto the artery wall. This triggers more white blood cells, continuing the cycle. Eventually, the artery becomes inflamed. The cholesterol plaque causes the muscle cells to enlarge and form a hard cover over the affected area. This is how this hard cover, called plaque, is created. It first hardens your arteries' walls and causes high blood pressure. It then evolves into the narrowing of and possible blocking of the blood flow through your arteries. If this happens to the arteries leading to your heart it may cause a heart attack. If the same happens to the arteries leading to your brain, it may cause a stroke.

Did You Know About The FDA Cholesterol "Update"?

In 2001, with the "helpful guidance of the pharmaceutical industry and its scientists", the FDA (Food and Drug Administration) "adjusted" its recommended guidelines for managing our cholesterol levels in the US. Prior to this change, the total dietary blood serum cholesterol count of less than 300 milligrams was considered acceptable. After this "new and improved" recommendation, only under 200 mg is considered acceptable. (JAMA 01;285:2486-2497).

If you're not paying attention, this change may seem to be of little importance to you, the average patient. But for the pharmaceutical companies, this new guideline instantly translated into additional billions of dollars of drug sales for them. Under the old rules, about 13 million people in this country "needed" (remember, these are "their" recommendations) to take cholesterol-lowering medications. Under the new ones, an additional 23 million people will now need to take these drugs. By helping adjust the federal guidelines by just a few points, pharmaceutical companies have almost tripled their cholesterol-lowering drug market. That's nice for them, not for us. Although they claim to do this for our own good, the increased sales are the more likely motivation. There is certainly a place for drugs in health care, but they are not the answer for all mankind's ills. What this means to you and me is that, although you should watch your cholesterol levels, you should also take these new levels with a grain of salt.

How to Read your "Updated" Cholesterol Report

In order for you to understand your blood panel result, you must first ask for it. Doctors will not necessarily give it to you. Read it carefully, and learn what the different levels are, and whether they are within the acceptable range.

What Levels of Total Cholesterol are Acceptable?

A total blood cholesterol level greater than 200 mg/dL, but less than 240 mg/dL, is considered by the American Heart Association (AHA) to be a moderately elevated cholesterol level. The AHA also considers this level to pose a borderline high risk to your health. Changes in diet and lifestyle are recommended for anyone with a total cholesterol level that falls into this range. A total blood cholesterol level greater than 240 mg/dL is considered to be high risk. This level carries with it a greater risk of heart attack, stroke, and coronary heart disease.

What are LDL and HDL?

Total cholesterol is not the only way - and not necessarily the best way - to evaluate your cholesterol status. Blood cholesterol can be broken down ("fractionated") into several types. These cholesterol types involve the various protein-containing molecules that transport cholesterol around the body. LDL (low-density lipoprotein) and HDL (high-density lipoprotein) are two of the best-studied transport molecules.

What Levels of LDL are Acceptable?

LDL carries cholesterol outward from the liver to the rest of the body tissue. This LDL cholesterol transporter is not capable of picking up cholesterol at various points around the body and bringing it back to the liver. The American Heart Association (AHA) recommends an LDL level of 100mg/dL or below as ideal. 130mg/dL is considered borderline high. Any LDL reading of 190mg/dL or above is considered very high.

What Levels of HDL are Acceptable?

The HDL transporter molecule is needed to carry out the "reverse" transport of cholesterol from tissues throughout the body back to the liver. Since this reverse transport of cholesterol back to the liver can help remove cholesterol from the bloodstream (and eventually from the body), HDL is considered a heart-protective transport molecule. Increasing your HDL level is most often a very helpful step in protecting the health of your heart.

An HDL level of 40-50 mg/dL is considered average for an adult male according to the American Heart Association (AHA). For adult women, the corresponding range is 50-60 mg/dL. If your HDL were below 40 mg/dL, the AHA would definitely consider that level too low.

What's a Good LDL/HDL Ratio?

Keeping your LDL/HDL ratio on the low side reduces your risk of heart problems. A ratio of 3:1 or below (no more than three times as much LDL as HDL) is almost always recommended. It takes a ratio of 2.3:1 or below to put you significantly below average risk.

What Should your Total Cholesterol/HDL Ratio Be?

It's also important not to confuse LDL/HDL ratio with total cholesterol/HDL ratio. This second type of ratio is also commonly used in cholesterol assessment. In the case of total cholesterol/HDL, a common goal is always to stay below 5:1 or between 0.00 and 4.44. But a total cholesterol/HDL ratio of 4:1 would be even better, and a ratio of 3.5:1 is described as optimal by the American Heart Association.

What are Triglycerides and what levels are acceptable?

Triglycerides levels should be below 160 mg/dL. In the human body, high levels of triglycerides in the bloodstream have been linked to atherosclerosis, and, by extension, the risk of heart disease and stroke. They are blood fats increased by sweets and alcohol. Your number should be between 35 and 160. The lower it is, the better. I personally feel that too much attention has been placed on total cholesterol levels, and not enough on triglycerides levels. I believe this country eats too much refined sugar in all its forms: not just the obvious like cookies and cakes but all forms of refined sugar, fructose, corn syrup and the worst of all, high fructose corn syrup (HFCS). These are found in everything from good ol' ketchup to salad dressings.

Statin Drugs Known Side Effects

Many people who take statins have suffered negative health consequences. The short list of known side effects caused by taking statin drugs include permanent damage to the liver, muscles and nervous system, as well as kidney failure. Statins frequently cause people to lose their memories or feel confused. Additional milder side effects include discomforts such as nausea, diarrhea, constipation; pains such as muscle aching or weakness, tingling or cramping in the legs, and inability to walk reasonable distances without resting. Mental difficulties such as sleep disruption, irritability, loss of mental clarity, mental confusion, possible amnesia, and neuropathy, as well as destruction of co-enzyme CoQ 10, an important enzyme in heart health support.

In my opinion, this is a big price to pay for trying to lower your cholesterol. Especially when changes in diet and lifestyle will automatically lower your cholesterol with no negative side effects. That is what this book will endeavor to do for you. Why should you unnecessarily suffer these nasty side effects when a tasty and healthy food alternative is available without too much effort?

Our Goal is to Lower LDL Levels and Increase HDL Levels with Food

Although I believe that in extreme cases, you may need drugs combined with lifestyle changes to help you lower your cholesterol levels to a reasonable level, I do not believe that drugs are the only answer. I know from experience that we can help ourselves through proper diet and lifestyle changes. There are three major ways to improve your cholesterol levels with diet. One, eat foods known to have a lowering effect on LDL (bad) cholesterol. Two, eat foods that boost your HDL (good) cholesterol. And three, eat foods loaded with antioxidants. All of these approaches are used in this book.

French Food to Lower Cholesterol?
Is that an Oxymoron?

For most people, lowering your cholesterol with French cuisine may seem to be a contradiction. When American people think of French cooking, they tend to think about rich food loaded with butter and cream, the way the old-fashioned "grande cuisine" used to be. Although there might still be a few French restaurants of that type out there, one major trend and one regional way of eating have moved modern French cuisine away from that stereotype.

For more than thirty years, the major trend in French cooking has been the Nouvelle Cuisine, created by a group of young and revolutionary chefs in the 1970's. The term was coined by the food critics Henri Gault and Christian Millaut to describe a trend started by Chef Fernand Point and his pupils and followers, a group that includes Michel Guerard, Roger Verge, Paul Bocuse, Alain Chapel and the pâtissier Gaston Lenotre. Their tenet was (and still is) that good food should not be loaded with dairy products or heavy sauces. Good food should stand on its own by the quality and utmost freshness of its ingredients. The Nouvelle Cuisine was lightly cooked, using the freshest meat, fowl, produce and fruits available locally and harvested only in season. The sauces were light, colorful and tasteful. The plate presentation was art in itself, colorful and well balanced. The serving plates were carefully chosen to be the canvas on which the food was presented. I was fortunate to have the opportunity to work in this environment when I worked for Roger Verge at the Moulin de Mougins, his famous restaurant in the South of France and for Gaston Lenotre in Paris and Houston.

Ideally, the Nouvelle Cuisine chef would go to the wholesale market early in the morning, pick the highest quality ingredients and create his menu based on what was available that day. It's a lot of work, but necessary for the creation of the freshest tasting and highest quality menu possible. That is why regional cuisine is so diverse in France: it gets its inspiration from the local ingredients only, not produce trucked or flown in from hundreds or thousands of miles away. It is also the healthiest way to eat. Freshly picked or harvested locally-grown food at the peak of freshness provides the most vitamins, minerals and live enzymes, which are beneficial to our bodies, on top of tasting great. The work of these luminaries of Nouvelle Cuisine inspires some of the recipes offered in this book.

The vast majority of the French population who could not afford to eat the rich Cuisine Bourgeoise (and there were a lot of us) always ate in a similar fashion. I still remember living on my grandparents' tiny, family-run farm. My "grand-père" was growing wheat for his landlord and was getting free lodging for his family, and a little money in exchange for his hard work. My "grand-mère", who was a big influence in my life, had to feed her family with pretty much what she could grow in her "potager" (food garden). So she had to know what to plant, how to take care of her garden and use what was available to feed her large family. She also raised her own chickens and rabbits for meat and eggs. Whatever product she could not produce herself, like the heavy "pain de campagne" (country-style bread) or "beurre frais" (fresh butter), she would trade at the farmers market with her own excess produce or rabbits. Although she was not what you would call a gourmet cook, she showed me that "la cuisine paysanne", made with simple but freshly picked ingredients, was indeed wonderful food. To honor her, I will include a few simple recipes that remind me of her.

Of course there has always been Cuisine de Santé offered in spas and health centers all over France. Typically, these were reserved for the well-to-do people who could afford to be pampered and follow the strict "régime" (diet) offered in these establishments. They would go there to "se refaire une santé" (regain their health) and go back to their unhealthy lifestyle for a while until they would return later to repair the damages created by the Cuisine Bourgeoise. They were "Health Vacations" for the rich. I will use a few of these recipes in this book to help you stay healthy without having to go to Eugenie Les Bains or Vittel, the famous spa towns of France.

French Mediterranean Cuisine: My Own Backyard

By far, my most important influence was my native environment. Although I was not born in the South of France, I got there as soon as I could, thanks to my family deciding to move from Paris to Nice to open a small hotel. What I did not realize at the time was that I landed in the heart of Mediterranean cuisine, world-renowned for its health attributes.

In the Lyon Diet Heart Study done between 1988 and 1992, people who had heart attacks were split into two groups. The first one was counseled to eat a Mediterranean diet, while the other received routine post-heart attack advice (watch your cholesterol, eat less saturated fats) and medications. After four years of follow-up, the group on the Mediterranean diet experienced 70 percent fewer heart attacks than the group getting the standard recommendations. That's about three times the reduction of risk of additional heart disease than achieved with statin drugs. They achieved a 45 percent reduction in the risk of dying from another heart attack. These results were so amazing that the study was stopped for ethical reasons: all the participants were told to follow the Mediterranean diet.

How did the French Mediterranean diet develop?

As in any other regional cuisine, the original Mediterranean diet evolved from the locally available ingredients: fish, fruits, vegetables, whole grains, olives and olive oil and nuts. As the Mediterranean region is typically hot and dry, the only animals raised in that region were goats, whose milk was used primarily for cheese. Up in the mountains, where grass could be found, sheep and lambs were raised for their wool and, for special occasions, their meat. Cows were not raised, as the dry climate produced insufficient grass. The main protein source was fish since most local economies were dependent on the sea.

When I was young, we could go to the Nice farmer's market and get the freshest fish from that morning's catch. One particular dish I enjoyed was called *poutine*, a simple dish made of tiny fishes tossed in flour and fried in olive oil. *Poutine* was served in newspaper cones, like French fries, and we picked them up whole with our greasy fingers, one by one, hot and crunchy and full of goodness, including omega-3 fatty acids and calcium from the bones. At that time I did not know anything about nutrition, but merely enjoyed them as a wonderful local dish and tradition.

You may have noticed that earlier I said "original" Mediterranean diet. My reason for that distinction is that as our world modernized and transportation and refrigeration became common, foods not usually found in our region became available to us as well as to the rest of the country. Cows meat and milk as well as "exotic" imported foods became available. As we wanted to become more sophisticated, we started to eat like the rest of the country and began to lose our wonderful and healthy diet. I still remember when industrialized food started to take over our local food. Our bread, the staple of the French diet, became this white, bland stick of gluten that became stale and inedible in a few hours. When I was a kid, my mom would send me every morning to the corner bakery to get our daily "baguettes" and "batards" still hot from the oven. They never made it home intact, as I loved to break off the crunchy ends and munch on them on my way back home. My mom did not like that, of course, but I figured that it was my reward for having to get out of bed early to go get the bread.

Nouvelle Cuisine Française

This state of affairs lasted from after World War II to the eighties. Then a group of young reactionary chefs, bakers and food professionals decided that enough was enough. They wanted to bring back our honored food culture and ancient traditions. So, all over the country, "artisans" bakers and chefs brought back our loved "slow" food the way we used to enjoy it, the traditional way. I suspect that the creation of the European Union, with a bunch of legislators in Brussels trying to regulate and codify how our food should be prepared, created a furious backlash in France (French folks are known to have a temper). We wanted our local culture and food back, and damn the legislators, we got it. This happened not only in France, but all over Europe as people realized that they wanted to save their regional traditions.

Welcome back *fougasse* (a Southern bread made with a touch of olive oil), *pissaladière* (a sort of pizza with only cooked onions and black Niçoise olives for topping), *socca* (a street-vendor dish made with garbanzo beans and olive oil), *soupe de poisons with rouille* (rock fish soup with saffron mayonnaise croutons), *daube Provençale* (meat stew cooked in red wine), *macarons aux amandes* (almond macaroons), and *salade Nicoise*, among myriad other regional specialties. They were never really lost as our elders were still saving their precious hand-written recipes in their kitchen drawers. I am proud to bring you some of these special dishes.

The Influence of Other Mediterranean Cuisines

As in many other countries, various historic and economic currents have influenced French culture. For example, after the Algerian war of independence, many of the French nationals who had emigrated there came back to France, bringing with them the dishes they used to cook in North Africa. There is a large contingent of these repatriates in Nice, my hometown. Also, as the "comté" of Nice kept being traded back and forth between France and Italy, depending on the current wars and occupations, our region became strongly influenced by Northern Italian food and culture. So there will be some of these Middle Eastern and Italian influences in the recipes I offer you.

French People and Their Food Philosophy

An important concept to keep in mind is that for French people, food is appreciated for its own goodness and the pleasure it can bring. Unlike Americans, the French typically do not care so much about nutrition. They do not count calories. They do not analyze every single molecule in their food to find out if it's good for them. If it's fresh, well prepared and tastes good, that's all that counts. Enjoying good food for the pleasure of eating is a way of life that should be learned and appreciated here in this country. We should not have to obsess about our food; healthy food can and should be one of life's pleasures.

My Healthy Food Philosophy

Now, in general, when you think of healthy food and special diets, you automatically think of over-boiled, limp and mushy vegetables, boring food of the type they serve in hospitals. If whatever brought you to the hospital in the first place does not kill you, the food they typically serve might finish you off - I am barely kidding. I have a personal experience to relate: when my son was hospitalized after a bad car accident and I saw what they were serving him as "food", I about jumped through the roof. That particular day, he was brought barely defrosted crinkled carrots and limp broccoli (I could also tell it was not fresh but frozen veggies), a flat-as-a-shoe-sole chicken-fried chicken (fried food? Yuk!) , coated with a gooey white gravy and let's not forget the finishing touch… green mint Jell-O. How did they expect my son to regain his strength with that kind of food?

When I protested, I was told this dreadful food was recommended by the hospital dietician. I tell you what! For the price they charged us for my son's hospital stay, they should have provided him with a 4-star meal. So I told the nurse (poor nurse, it was not her fault, of course) that from now on, my wife and I would bring home-cooked food and additional herbal supplements to aid in his recovery. Of course, she told us it was against policy but at that point, I did not care. She understood. Although it might have gotten her into trouble, she allowed us to bring our son healthy home-cooked meals and I believe my son's recovery was accelerated because of it.

Healthy food should Taste and Look Good

As a French-born and French-trained chef, taste and presentation are of utmost importance to me. Let us consider presentation: we are visual creatures. If the food looks appealing, we are more likely to give it a try. But it has to deliver on its promise. If your food tastes as good as it looks, then it pleases all our senses and becomes a pleasant experience we will want to repeat. This goes for healthy food prepared at home as much as any restaurant dish. That is what I'm trying to accomplish with the recipes I am providing in this book: my goal is to encourage you to eat healthy food because it tastes and looks so good.

A Note about Nutritional Values

I suppose some of you may expect to see a nutritional analysis with every recipe. I decided not to include them as it would go against the spirit of this program. I want this to be all about eating healthy food for the pleasure of it. What I do not want is for you to obsess about counting calories, fats and beans. The recipes are designed to be both flavorful and healthy. Trust them to provide that and enjoy the journey into better health.

Healthy Food Preparations

In order to keep the good qualities of the food you buy at the market, it is important not to damage it with the cooking techniques you use. Although I am not a raw foodist, I believe many foods should be eaten either raw or lightly cooked to preserve their nutritional qualities. Raw food contains a lot of vitamins and minerals that are important to our health. It does not make sense to destroy these qualities by over-processing or over-cooking.

- Raw food: preparing raw food preserves all the vital nutrients of the quality food you have taken pains to choose. It retains all the vitamins, minerals, antioxidants, phytonutrients and enzymes necessary to keep your body healthy. I am not purely a raw food advocate but I do believe that we should eat at least half of our food raw.

- Light steaming: I prefer to use steaming instead of boiling to lightly cook vegetables. Light cooking can tenderize asparagus or artichokes and make them easier to digest, or bring out the carotenoids locked in raw carrots and tomatoes. You should steam for 5 to 7 minutes at the most to keep your vegetables al dente (crunchy) and full of nutrients.

- Blanching: To blanch vegetables, bring a pot of water to a rolling boil, drop them in the water, bring the water back to a boil and cook for no longer than one minute or until they turn bright green . Take your vegetables out the boiling water with a slotted spoon and drop in iced water to stop the cooking process and keep your vegetables crunchy. There will be a little more loss of vitamins by this method, but it still is a very healthy way to cook.

- Simmering: This technique relates mostly to soups and stews where the food is cooked for a longer time at a lower temperature. This method allows the food to tenderize while blending all the wonderful flavors together. Many of the nutrients are preserved in the broth or the sauce.

- Broth poaching: This is one of my favorite ways to cook asparagus and other vegetables. Pour a small amount of a good quality broth (vegetable, fish, beef or chicken according to the dish) in the bottom of a stainless steel pan or skillet; bring to a simmer. Place your vegetables in the broth and cook for 3-4 minutes on one side; turn your vegetables over and finish to cook for another 3-4 minutes, according to the size of your vegetables. Drizzle with a freshly made vinaigrette or olive oil and lemon juice, sea salt and ground pepper and voila! A quick, simple and healthy dish.

- Quick sautéing or Stir Fry: It's no secret that I do not like deep fried cooking method (see below), but a quick sautéing is an acceptable way of cooking if you follow my advice. Do not overheat your oil; if it smokes, it means it is oxidized and damaged. Throw it away and start over. An easy way to find out when your oil is hot enough to cook is to sprinkle your oil pan with a little water. When it "sings" (that's the way I like to call it. Some people prefer to say "sizzles"), I know the oil is hot enough to cook. Quick sautéing is a good cooking method for a yummy omelet or sautéed vegetables. The oil will bring out the carotenoids locked in their raw state. Make sure to *never* reuse the oil.

- Quick Broiling: I learned this method in the restaurant business. I also discovered by accident that it is a very healthy way to cook some foods, especially fatty fish like salmon. To quick broil, preheat your oven at the Broil level; place a glazed cast iron or stainless steel skillet in the oven. (I recommend Le Creuset, my favorite pots and pans for the past 30 years.) Allow the pan/skillet to heat for at least 10 minutes; take it out with oven mittens and place your fish or meat in it; put it quickly back in the oven and cook for a few minutes. As a matter of fact, that is the only way I will cook my fish and meat nowadays. It is quick (3 to 5 minutes depending how thick your piece of salmon is), it preserves the healthy qualities of your food (in salmon's case, its omega-3 fatty acids) while offering a pleasant mouth feel. Your food is crunchy on the outside while moist on the inside.

- <u>"En papillote"</u> This is a method rarely used outside of the restaurant business, as it can be involving. You create a parchment pocket where you place all the ingredients you want to cook, fold the paper over on itself tightly so it forms a sort of envelope, and you cook it all in the oven. The advantage of this method is that all the ingredients simmer and flavor each other. It is a wonderful method, but you might want to try this on a weekend when you have more time.

Unhealthy Food Preparations

Techniques you will never see in this book are: deep fat frying, grilling, barbecuing (sorry Texas), high temperature cooking and worst of all, microwaving.

- Deep Fat Frying: Even though French fries are cooked with this method (and I do admit that, a couple of times a year, I will indulge my love of French fries. Hey, I never claimed I was perfect!), in the long term, it is a very unhealthy way of cooking your food. First of all, most likely, vegetable shortening (a trans-fatty acid known to clog your arteries worse than saturated fats) will be used. To make things worse, that fat is heated over and over. Even when it's filtered at night, small food particles and flour coating has been cooked all day in that cauldron of hell. That creates carcinogens that may bring you an assorted menu of cancers. Even if high smoking point oil is used, the repeated heating process will oxidize these oils and damage your health. Never, never, NEVER eat at fast food establishments (notice, I did not use the term restaurant) as their food is always fried and very unhealthy for you. If you're curious to know more, please watch the documentary "Supersize Me" by Morgan Spurlock. This movie will open your eyes to the dangers of fried food. If you must deep fry your food, do it at home and be very careful to not overheat your oil, and never reuse that oil again.

- Grilling: Although grilling is touted as a healthier way of cooking than frying, it is not. Unfortunately, grilling creates a form of a toxin called heterocyclic amines (HAs), which are well researched carcinogens. Another compound created by direct flame grilling is called polycyclic aromatic hydrocarbons (PAHs), which might be as equally harmful. That charred flavor you love in your grilled food is not that friendly to you. Beware!

- Barbecuing: I know I'm going to make enemies here in Texas, but I must be honest with you: barbecuing is as bad as grilling when it comes to the creation of unhealthy compounds. When the free amino acids from protein, creatine (or creatinine), and the sugar in the barbeque sauce used to baste and flavor the meat combine, they create our old friends the heterocyclic amines (HAs).

- <u>High Temperature Cooking</u>: Research conducted by the Mount Sinai Medical Hospital found that foods cooked at high temperatures contain a greater amount of compounds called advanced glycation end products (AGEs) that cause more tissue damage and inflammation than foods cooked at lower temperatures. That is why I recommend the lower cooking temperatures techniques you can find above.

- <u>Microwaving</u>: In my opinion, this is the worst of all cooking methods and the most dangerous to our health. Did you know that the Soviet Union banned the use of microwave ovens in 1976? And, here we go, eating food cooked in a way that destroys all the healthy attributes of our food and even of water.

Microwaves are a form of electromagnetic energy, like light waves or radio waves. Every microwave oven contains a magnetron, which creates microwaves of energy. When you push that button on your microwave oven, the microwaves generated from the magnetron bombard your food, agitate your food's molecules – especially water - a million times per second, creating friction which heats your food. So far, so good. Unfortunately, it has been found that this same friction deforms the food molecules and makes them dangerous to our health.

In 1992, Dr. Hertel, a Swiss scientist, was the first scientist to conceive of and carry out a quality clinical study of the effects microwaved nutrients have on the blood and physiology of the human body. His small but well controlled study showed the degenerative force produced in microwave ovens and the food processed in them. The scientific conclusion showed that microwave cooking changed the nutrients in the food. Changes also took place in the participants' blood that could cause deterioration in the human system. Hemoglobin levels decreased and overall white cell levels and cholesterol levels increased. Lymphocytes, the foot soldiers of the immune system, decreased, opening the way for disease.

My mother never trusted her food to this newfangled electronic gizmo. I never cook with it and neither should you. Throw the darned thing away. You will be better off in the long run. You don't have to take my word for it. For your own sake, please do your own research if you need further convincing.

Physical Exercise

What? You did not think I was going to talk about exercise? Well, here it is, but you don't need to worry. In my opinion, exercise does not have to be painful or strenuous. Honestly, as a Frenchman, my focus is not on using exercise to counter the effects of a bad diet; I would prefer you eat healthfully and skip the exercise. After all, I am from the South of France. We have a reputation for laziness to uphold. But even I do a *little* exercise. Nothing to brag about, but enough to stay healthy. Notice, I did not say to get strong, beefy or bulky. I have no intention of breaking any world records.

Walking

Walking is one form of light exercise that I endorse. Not speed walking, but walking. Typically I take a 20 minute walk every day (you're welcome to make it twice a day, but my job is physical enough. I'm pretty tired by the end of the day). Start slowly, bring up your heart rate gently and increase the pace as you're moving along. Towards the end, slow down a little to bring your heart rate back down and Voila! You're done. What I try to do is focus on my breathing and not on my speed. Again, this is not a race. Walking will massage all your internal organs and move your lymph fluids around which helps in toxin elimination through the skin.

I prefer to do it early in the morning when it's still cool and the birds are waking up. If you have an hour lunch break, it's a good idea to do your walk after lunch so you do not fall asleep at your desk. If it is too hot outside, walk up and down your office building stairs or get to the nearest shopping mall and walk around in air conditioned comfort, just no shopping, OK? Or you could wait until after dinner and walk your dog at the same time. Walking will help you sleep a lot better too. Find a time and place to walk that works for you. The whole idea is to enjoy it, not dread it.

My Not-so-secret Other Form of Exercise

All my friends can tell you: I love to dance. Dance is a wonderful form of exercise and it's fun. How can you beat that? Whenever possible, I take one dance class a week, break a sweat and burn off a few calories. The most important part is that I move, and move a lot. Right now, I'm into salsa (not the sauce) and I love it. When I have a partner, we go out to dance at least once a week. You'd be surprised how much exercise you can get while dancing and you don't even realize it. That's the whole idea of doing a sport/exercise you enjoy. You're making yourself healthier and don't even have to think about it.

Do What you Enjoy Most and you Will be Happier and Healthier

Besides these two simples ideas, feel free to take up any physical activity you enjoy. If you love tennis but have not practiced for a while, try it again at a lower level and work your way up gently. That's what my brother did: after years of enjoying his wife's wonderful cooking, he started to look like a stuffed turkey. Actually his nieces used to tease him and call him "tonton gros ventre" (big-bellied uncle). After taking this "verbal abuse" for a few years, he decided to go back to his favorite sport, tennis, and started to work on improving his game, one match at a time. Now in his late forties, he boasts proudly of "kicking butts" of people half his age. So there's hope for you too! If you love it, you will do it.

Another Healthy Non-Exercise you May Want to Try

Another form of non-exercise that is good for you is meditation or quiet prayer. I started doing this a few years ago on a good friend's recommendation, and it works. Not only can it connect you to a higher power (whichever that might be for you), you also center and calm yourself before and after your workday. Some people say it's even better than taking a 20-minute power nap, because the brain waves generated by meditation offer better rest than sleeping for such a short time. For me quiet prayer is what works. It prepares me for the day and helps me return to calmness in the evening. My favorite recommendation would be meditating in the morning before a busy day and a walk in the evening, after dinner to help your digestion. Or you can do it the other way around. Try it and see which way works best for you; either way it will do you good.

Is There Going to be Work Involved?

Yes, for some of you this will involve a complete lifestyle change. You will have to change your shopping habits. Some of you will have to change the way you think about food, not just as a way to survive from meal to meal but another way to enjoy life as you enjoy your favorite hobby. Maybe it will become your new hobby, you never know! Becoming healthier is a very good incentive to get started. If you're lucky, your spouse knows how to cook and will be glad to help you regain a healthy lifestyle with guidance from this book. If not, it's a perfect opportunity for the two of you to start a new hobby together. It is always easier when you face a new situation hand in hand. Bonne chance!

If you have a hard time cooking from scratch, I suggest you take a few basic cooking classes. Nowadays, classes are available everywhere. In Austin we are very lucky, we can take cooking classes at Whole Foods Market, Central Market, the Culinary Academy of Austin, the Texas Culinary Academy and a multitude of other locations. Actually, I teach classes in some of these locations, so drop in sometime if you feel like it. I am sure cooking classes are available no matter where you live. You don't need to be a gourmet cook to prepare these recipes; I tried to keep them simple and easy to understand. I also suggest quick and healthy cooking techniques so you do not have to spend hours in the kitchen. That would defeat the purpose. The last thing I want is to discourage you from starting this journey to better heath.

My Secret to Happy Eating and Good Heath is Now Your Secret

My secret is for you to be conscious and aware of your food choices, but not to obsess about it. Try to make daily progress, and if you cheat once in a while, it's okay as long as you understand why you're doing it and don't make yourself feel guilty about it. Me, I do eat French cheese once in a while on special occasions. Of course, I'm French. Cheese is running through my veins (not really). Eat a variety of fresh and healthy foods. Eat small servings and don't overcook your food. Will you join me in this health-rediscovery adventure? **A Votre Santé and Bon Appétit!**

Foods That Affect Your Cholesterol Levels

Why I feel this Book is Important for you

Although I believe that in extreme cases, you may need drugs combined with lifestyle changes to help you lower your cholesterol levels to as reasonable level, I do not believe that drugs are the only answer. I firmly believe that we can help ourselves by watching what we eat and the quality of the food we ingest. So let's talk about the way to reduce our LDL and triglycerides levels and increase our HDL levels through proper diet and lifestyle changes.

Our Goal is to Lower LDL Levels and Increase HDL Levels with Food

How do we do that? To lower LDL, we need to eliminate or avoid the consumption of the damaging foods described below. To increase HDL we need to eat more of the foods good for us. It's that easy. I will attempt to help you understand how you can do it on your own (with a little help from me).

Foods That Increase Your LDL (bad) Cholesterol Levels

Hydrogenated Fats: Margarine and Shortening

For decades, nutritionists, physicians, and health publications have sold the public on the idea that margarine is "heart smart". It's even served in hospitals, for Pete's sake! Margarine is a product of hydrogenation and is far more dangerous to your health than butter. The fats it contains are not compatible with human body chemistry. They have a higher melting point than body temperature, which means they will not melt inside your body, so they circulate in your bloodstream as a solid fat. Studies from as early as the 1950s have shown that these man-made, hardened oils are dangerous.

During the process of hydrogenation, hydrogen is "bubbled" through liquid oils. The extra hydrogen atoms turn unsaturated liquid oils into saturated fat, producing some pretty strange fat molecules that aren't naturally found in the human food chain. Hydrogenated fats alter the normal production of fatty-like hormones called prostaglandins. Over 100 different varieties of prostaglandins are known to exist, and preliminary studies indicate they have links to blood pressure, free-radical scavenging, transmission of nerve impulses, inflammatory reactions, blood clotting, and even cancer.

These unusual fat molecules also change the melting points of substances. While unrefined, unsaturated fats melt at around 55°F or less, hydrogenated fats won't melt until around 112°F. The fact that they don't smoke or burn at higher temperatures makes them ideal to use in deep-frying (ideal for the owner of the fast-food franchise and the heart surgeon, that is.) They don't absorb flavor from food, so chicken, fish, and onion rings can all be fried in the same grease. And best of all, the customer can't taste any difference when the oil becomes rancid. This last feature makes hydrogenated oils a popular ingredient for cookies and crackers that need a long shelf life.

Saturated Fats from Animal Sources

Excessive dietary intake of foods rich in saturated fat and cholesterol, which are found primarily in meat, particularly red meat, and other animal products, is strongly associated with increased risk of atherosclerosis and heart disease. Please note the word *excessive*. If you eat a reasonable amount (4 ounces per serving per day) of grass-fed beef or free-range bison, I don't believe you will hurt yourself. You have to remember that the vast majority of the meat we find in the supermarket is raised on corn feed which increases the amount of polyunsaturated fats in the meat (yellow fat). Since industrial polyunsaturated fats are oxidative in your body, they will damage your arteries thus increasing cholesterol deposits. So my recommendation is quality grass-fed meat, in moderation.

Avoid Fried Foods. Remember that even the best oils turn from cis-fatty acids (healthy) to trans-fatty acids (unhealthy) when overheated. If you do end up frying something, don't heat the oil high enough to make it smoke. Use monounsaturated, non-hydrogenated oils for sautéing, such as olive oil, macadamia oil and coconut oil. Do not reuse cooking oils.

Alain's cooking tips
When I pan-fry my own omelet (my treat for Sunday's brunch), I heat up half extra virgin olive oil mixed with half organic butter. When the butter "sings" or sizzles your fats have reached the ideal temperature for frying. If the butter burns, throw away everything, wash the pan and start over. Better that, than ingesting damaged fats.

Refined Sugars: The Good, The Bad and The Ugly

Can your life be any sweeter than it is? Or can refined sugar make your life miserable? Maybe you should think about it before you answer this one. One of the greatest joys of life is eating, and sweeteners make many foods taste delicious! It is said that the average American consumes 150 pounds of assorted sweeteners per year. An American child consumes twice as much, mostly in the form of soft drinks. The most widely used sweeteners are conventional white sugar and high fructose corn syrup. Both are highly processed sweeteners and are not recommended by this guide, as they offer no benefits to the health-conscious and environmentally responsible consumer.

A Little Sugar Here and There will not Kill Me, Right?

I know we all tend to be attracted to the bad boys or girls. But this is a choice that will affect you for much longer than a broken heart. Sugar may actually break it in a more final way if you can't resist the temptation of its sweet embrace. What I am talking about? Well let's start with hypoglycemia, possibly going up to adult-onset diabetes (Type II) and all the way to serious heart disease and all its miseries.

According to the well-respected nutritionist Nancy Appleton, Ph. D., sugar affects our bodies negatively in 146 ways. While I will limit myself to the few related to our cholesterol problem, if you're curious about overall negative effect on our health, I strongly suggest you buy her books or check her website: http://www.nancyappleton.com/.

Here are the few we should be aware of:

- Sugar can produce a significant rise in triglycerides.
- Sugar reduces high-density lipoproteins or HDL (good) cholesterol.
- Sugar contributes to obesity.
- Sugar can increase cholesterol.
- Sugar can cause atherosclerosis.
- Sugar can promote an elevation of low-density lipoproteins or LDL (bad) cholesterol.
- Sugar can cause platelet adhesiveness.

- Sugar is an addictive substance.

Some nutritionists will say sugar, no matter where it comes from, is bad for you. Although I agree with them, I am also fully aware that the vast majority of people will not go without. If, with the following advice, I can steer you towards the healthier forms of sugar and make you aware of the "bad" and "ugly" sweeteners, I think I've done my job. Ultimately, my advice is to reduce your sugar intake as much as possible. Sorry, but as much as I'd like to, I can't be there to crack the whip. It's up to you.

The Good: Natural Sweeteners

There is a broad spectrum of healthy sweeteners to choose from, and they vary in degrees of processing and nutrition. Raw and minimally processed sweeteners generally contain more nutrition than the highly processed alternatives. Organic sweeteners have the added benefit of being grown and processed in a way that is not only healthier for us but for the environment as well. Look for products that have an organic certification to be sure that you are purchasing products that have been grown and processed without using harmful chemicals, pesticides, or herbicides. These organic practices help protect our environment by eliminating polluting chemicals from entering our soil, groundwater, plants, and atmosphere.

Because any one sweetener type may or may not be organic, this guide will not distinguish between "organic molasses" and "molasses". It will only describe the characteristics of sweeteners as a whole. In alphabetical order:

Agave Nectar
A sweetener naturally extracted from the Americana Agave (a cactus-like plant native to Mexico). Because of its low glycemic index (40% lower than sugar), agave nectar is absorbed slowly into your bloodstream. It also provides vitamins and minerals not found in processed sweeteners.

Vegans in particular commonly use agave syrup to replace honey in recipes. It is also a very effective sweetener for cold beverages such as iced tea as, unlike sugar and honey, it dissolves readily in cold liquids. Raw agave nectar also has a mild, neutral taste. Agave nectar is an acceptable sweetener for people with hypoglycemia, as long as you control its usage. I would be cautious to recommend it for people with type 1 or type 2 diabetes, as its glycemic index is 27.

Barley Malt
Barley malt is made by fermenting grain. The fermenting bacteria convert the grain starches into simple and complex sugars and the final product consists of 40% complex carbohydrates. Its glycemic index is 75.

Concentrated Fruit Juices
Concentrated fruit juices are highly refined sources of sugar that contain very little of the nutrients present in fresh fruit and none of the fiber that balances blood sugar. These sweeteners bear little resemblance to the fruit from which they are derived. It is recommended to use organic frozen fruit juice instead of fruit syrups, which are even more concentrated.

Date "Sugar"
Date sugar is made by pulverizing dried dates. It is not refined like sugar and, therefore, contains the nutrients and minerals found in dates. Date sugar also contains fiber.

Honey
Honey is a sweet, viscous fluid made by honeybees from the nectar of flowering plants. Flavors vary depending upon the plant source from which the nectar is derived. The worker bee transforms the sucrose of nectar into the simple sugars fructose and glucose. Honey is sweeter than sugar, has more calories than sugar and raises the blood sugar even more than white sugar. Raw honey is said to have medicinal benefits and contains enzymes and small amounts of minerals and B-complex vitamins. Honey can be purchased in liquid and granular forms. I suggest you use only honey collected locally and minimally processed, not the honey bear type. I use creamy honey from Premium Research Labs in Round Rock, TX. (Note: It has been suggested that honey should not be given to children under the age of 18 months because their digestive tracts and immune systems are not yet developed enough for bacteria that may be present in honey.) Its glycemic index is 83.

Maple syrup

Maple syrup is a sweetener made from the sap of maple trees. In Canada and the United States it is most often eaten with pancakes, waffles, French toast, cornbread or ice cream. It is sometimes used as an ingredient in baking, the making of candy, preparing desserts, or as a sugar source and flavoring agent in making beer. Sucrose is the most prevalent sugar in maple syrup.

When you want to satisfy your sweet tooth, don't forget to consider using maple syrup, which contains fewer calories and a higher concentration of minerals than honey. It is available throughout the year in your local supermarket. It has a glycemic index of 54 while white sugar is 95.

Molasses

Blackstrap molasses is the final product of the sugar-making process. Blackstrap molasses contains more of the vitamins, minerals, and trace elements (iron, potassium, calcium and magnesium) found naturally in the sugar cane plant, making it more nutritious than most other sweeteners. Its glycemic index is 65.

Barbados molasses is another type of molasses, but unlike blackstrap molasses, it is one of the first products produced in the sugar-making process. As one of the first products produced, Barbados molasses is lighter and sweeter than blackstrap because it has a higher sucrose content than blackstrap. It is an excellent choice when the blackstrap variety is too strong or not sweet enough. Its glycemic index is 69.

Rice Syrup

Rice syrup is a sweetener prepared by culturing rice with enzymes to break down the starches, straining off the liquid, and cooking it to the desired consistency. Brown rice syrup contains 50% soluble complex carbohydrates, which take from two to three hours to be digested, resulting in a steady supply of energy. This syrup can be evaporated to form a rice syrup powder. Its glycemic index is 20.

Sucanat

Sucanat is the only sugar cane product of its kind, is made by keeping together the two products that typical sugar processing tries to separate - sugar and molasses. The initial pressing of the sugar cane plant contains all of the elements of both sugar and molasses. Through the sugar making process, these two products are separated. All of the nutritional benefits of the sugar cane plant remain with the molasses leaving sugar as "empty calories."

In making Sucanat, two key things are accomplished. First, unlike brown sugar where molasses is simply added back to sugar for color, the molasses and sugar are kept together from the beginning of the process. This creates a dry sweetener product with the vitamins, minerals and trace elements of the sugar cane plant and a lower sucrose level than refined white and brown sugar. Second, the crystals that are formed are actually bonded naturally, forming a granule that is easier to blend with the other ingredients and creates a smoother texture in baked goods. Its glycemic index is the same as white sugar, 95.

Unrefined sugar

Unrefined sugar is made from sugar cane juice that is released by pressing sugar cane stalks. It is different from refined sugar in that it is typically 50% less processed and therefore contains slightly more molasses than refined sugar. Unrefined sugar has a sucrose level in the range of 99.2% - 99.5% as compared to refined sugar, which has a higher sucrose level of 99.9%. It is usually called Raw Sugar or Turbinado Sugar, or even Raw Turbinado Sugar. Its glycemic index is the same as white sugar, 95.

Naturally Occurring Alternative Sweeteners

Stevia

Stevia Rebaudiana is an herb in the *Compositae* family that grows as a small shrub in parts of Paraguay and Brazil. The glycosides in its leaves make it incredibly sweet, a property that is unique among the nearly 300 species of stevia plants. Stevia has been used to sweeten beverages and medicines since Pre-Columbian times. A scientist named Antonio Bertoni first recorded its usage by native tribes in 1887.

This is my favorite sweetener for people with blood sugar problems such as diabetes or hypoglycemia. It's an all-natural product with zero calories, zero carbs and a score of zero on the glycemic index. It does not affect your blood sugar level. My favorite brand is SweetLeaf Stevia. There's a slight aftertaste.

Dragon Herbs SweetFruit Drops

Another natural sweetener extracted from a plant is *Guilin* SweetFruit extract. It is the tincture of *glucoside,* from the Chinese herb/fruit Luo Han Guo (*Momordica grosvenori*). It is a sweetening product that has virtually no effect on blood sugar level. It is up to 300 times sweeter than refined sugar and has just 5 percent of the calories of sugar. Luo Han Guo Glucoside is a stable non-fermentable substance with high sweetness and low heat. It can be used to sweeten all kinds of drinks and food as a substitute for sugar. It is an ideal sweetening agent for people with hypoglycemia or Diabetes. For people that do not care for Stevia's aftertaste, this product has a clean finish. No glycemic index available.

Fructooligosaccharides (FOS)

They occur naturally in some grains and vegetables. They are known as a food that encourages the growth of beneficial intestinal bacteria. (They don't encourage *C. albicans*.) They have several additional advantages. FOS are sucrose molecules to which 1-3 additional fructose molecules are attached. Because of this, they taste sweet but are too large to be digested as a sugar. Therefore, they have no caloric effect and no effect on blood sugar levels. Although this substance is widely used as a sweetener in Japan (where it has been popular for nearly a decade), it is currently too expensive in this country to be used as a common sweetener. Hopefully, this will change in the near future.

Lo Han

The newest entry in the sugar alternatives is named Lo Han Kuo or Lo Han for short. It is extracted from a fruit grown in China. Lo Han is so low in calories that one serving has no measurable caloric value. It also has an incredibly low glycemic index. It does not cause sweet cravings and has no influence on insulin production and fat storage. Lo Han does not raise blood sugar level and is safe for most diabetics and hypoglycemic people (if you're' not sure, please double-check with your doctor).

Best of all, it tastes great. Its flavor is slightly more rounded and more complex than white sugar, a bit like maple syrup. It does not have the slightly bitter aftertaste that Stevia does. Lo Han can be used in cereals, tea, or wherever you would use white sugar. Be careful, as Lo Han is 10-15 times as sweet as sugar. A little goes a long way. Although Lo Han's price has dropped recently and is now more affordable, it is still pricier than most alternative sweeteners. Lo Han is sold by TriMedica as SlimSweet and a few other makers as well. If you look hard enough, you can even find beverages sweetened with Lo Han. No glycemic index available.

Substitution in Recipes

Substituting healthy sweeteners for conventional white sugar in recipes is easy! You'll enjoy the wonderful textures and rich flavors that healthy sweeteners add to your favorite recipes. When you find the perfect substitute, cross out sugar and white flour and write in the healthy or organic substitute.

Substitution Chart
Commonly Used Sweeteners Equivalent to 1 Cup of White Sugar

Sucanat: 1 cup

Unrefined Sugar: 1 cup

Date Sugar: 1 cup

Barley Malt: 1 ½ cup-Reduce liquids by 1-2 tablespoons

Brown Rice Syrup: 1 cup powder

Molasses: ½ to ¾ cup

Concentrated Fruit Juices: Varies

Honey: ½ cup. Reduce liquid by ½ cup & Temperatures by 25 ¼ F

The Bad: Corn Syrup, High Fructose Corn Syrup (HFCS) and Refined Fructose

Corn Syrup

Corn syrup is commercial glucose made from chemically purified cornstarch with everything removed except the starch. Most corn syrup has sugar syrup added to it because glucose is only half as sweet as white sugar. It is highly refined and absorbs into the bloodstream very quickly, which is very bad for hypoglycemic and diabetic people.

Refined Fructose

Fructose is a natural sugar found in plants and fruits, but generally is a highly refined product made from cornstarch. It is very low in nutrients. For some people there are disadvantages to consuming large amounts of fructose: increased LDL cholesterol levels, increased uric-acid levels in the blood, and higher triglyceride levels. However, it is absorbed more slowly in the gastro-intestinal tract than glucose, producing only a slight insulin response, resulting in smaller fluctuations in blood-sugar levels.

The primary reason fructose is used commercially in foods and beverages is because of its relative sweetness. It is the sweetest of all naturally occurring carbohydrates. Fructose is 1.73 times sweeter than sucrose.

Consuming glucose starts a cascade of biochemical reactions. It increases production of insulin by the pancreas, which enables sugar in the blood to be transported into cells, where it can be used for energy. It increases production of leptin, a hormone that helps regulate appetite and fat storage, and it suppresses production of another hormone made by the stomach, ghrelin, that helps regulate food intake. It has been theorized that when ghrelin levels drop, as they do after eating carbohydrates composed of glucose, hunger declines.

Fructose is like a wolf in sheep's clothes. It appears to behave more like fat with respect to the hormones involved in body weight regulation. Fructose doesn't stimulate insulin secretion. It doesn't increase leptin production nor suppress production of ghrelin. That suggests that consuming a lot of fructose, like consuming too much fat, could contribute to weight gain. In other words, refined fructose is as bad as refined sucrose or white sugar.

High Fructose Corn Syrup is any of a group of corn syrups which have undergone enzymatic processing in order to increase their fructose content, which are then mixed with pure corn syrup (100% glucose) to reach their final form. According to one study, the average American consumes nearly 70 pounds of HFCS per annum, marking HFCS as a major contributor to the rising rates of obesity in the last generation. For more details on fructose and high fructose corn syrup, please go to:
http://www.westonaprice.org/modernfood/highfructose.html

The Ugly: Artificial Sweeteners. How Sweet are They?

The FDA regulates artificial sweeteners as food additives, which must be approved as safe before they can be marketed. To date, the FDA has approved five artificial sweeteners. But just how safe are they?

Acesulfame Potassium or Acesulfame-K (Sunett, Sweet One)

A combination of potassium, sulfur, nitrogen, carbon, and hydrogen. The Center for Science in the Public Interest recommends that people avoid use of acesulfame-K due to lack of testing concerns.

Aspartame (NutraSweet, Equal)

A combination of two amino acids - aspartic acid and phenylalanine. Because of the phenylalanine component, aspartame carries a risk for people with the rare genetic disorder phenylketonuria. The Center for Science in the Public Interest recommends that people - especially young children - avoid use of aspartame due to cancer concerns. Therefore, it is not recommended for use by pregnant or lactating women. Equal contains aspartame, dextrose, and maltodextrin. When the sweetener aspartame is digested, its methyl ester bond is broken down into methanol, which further degrades into formaldehyde, although a minute amount. According to **DORway to Discovery,** aspartame mimics symptoms or worsens the following diseases: fibromyalgia, arthritis, multiple sclerosis (MS), Parkinson's disease, lupus, multiple chemical sensitivities (MCS), diabetes and diabetic complications, epilepsy, Alzheimer's disease, birth defects, chronic fatigue syndrome, lymphoma, Lyme disease, attention deficit disorder (ADD), panic disorder, depression and other psychological disorders.

Neotame

A derivative of the dipeptide composed of the following amino acids: aspartic acid and phenylalanine. While some of the components are the same as aspartame, products made with neotame require no special labeling for phenylketonuria. Owned by NutraSweet and not marketed to the consumer in bulk or packet form. The Center for Science in the Public Interest indicates that the additive appears to be safe. **DORway to Discovery** would differ with this assessment.

Saccharin (Sweet'N Low, Sweet Twin, Necta Sweet, Sugar Twin)

A chemical derived from coal tar, a compound of carbon, nitrogen, oxygen, and sulfur atoms. Controversial since the 1970's, when studies linked saccharin to cancer. Most long-term animal studies, however, have found no cancer-causing effects from saccharin consumption. On December 15, 2000, Congress passed legislation to remove the warning label that had been required on saccharin-sweetened foods and beverages since 1977. The National Toxicology Program has removed saccharin from its list of cancer-causing substances. On its website, the Center for Science in the Public Interest still recommends that people avoid use of saccharin due to cancer concerns. However, Dr. Jane Starr Hull considers saccharin the safest of the artificial packet sweeteners.

Sucralose (Splenda)

Its manufacturer, McNeil Nutritionals, long advertised Splenda as being "made from sugar, so it tastes like sugar." In fact, the sweetener is a synthetic chemical made by chemically reacting sugar (sucrose) with chlorine. Sucralose is not absorbed from the digestive tract, so it adds no calories to consumed food. In addition, sucralose does not increase blood sugar levels. The Center for Science in the Public Interest indicates that the additive appears to be safe. Prevention notes that there is little research on sucralose use so it is advisable to limit use until long-term effects are known.

The bottom line is that artificial sweeteners are just that, artificial. We are probably all better served by choosing natural sweeteners and training our taste buds to savor less sweet foods and drinks.

Foods that are Good for your HDL (good) Cholesterol

First, the Old Fat Controversy: Is it Good or Bad for Us?

The fat issue is so complex that whole books have been written on the subject (one I like is: **Fats That Can Save Your Life** by Robert Herdmann, Ph.D.) I will try to give you a shorter explanation as well as my personal opinions on this subject. First, the "good" fats:

There are different "families" of fats. They all have different effects on your health. The one you probably think you know the most about is:

- **Saturated fats**: Saturated fats mostly come from animals (contained in animal meat and fat such as lard and from animal products like butter) but can also come from plants like coconut. They are called saturated because they become solid at room temperature. In my opinion, if you use a good quality saturated fat (see raw butter and pure coconut oil below) and use a moderate amount, saturated fats can actually be good for you. My secret is quality and moderation.

- **Unsaturated fats**. They come in two sub-families

    - **Monounsaturated fats**: Also called omega-9 fatty acids also called oleic acid can be found in nuts, olives and olive oil and avocado. It is known to lower heart attack risk and arteriosclerosis, and can aid in cancer prevention. Always remember to get your omega-9s from natural and unprocessed sources. That's the only way they should be consumed. See more info below in the olive oil and macadamia oil paragraph.

    - **Polyunsaturated fats**: They come in two types:

        o **The omega-3 fatty acids**. There are 3 different types, all considered to be essential fatty acids (EFAs).

            ▪ **Animal source**: Omega-3s can be found in animal products such as fatty fish and fish oil. In this case, they are formed from two special fatty acids: DHA (*docosahexaenoic acid*) and EPA (*eicosapentaenoic acid*) are the most easily assimilated and beneficial to our body. These are considered to be the highest quality of omega-3, as our body can utilize them faster to keep itself functioning properly.

Frequent consumption of wild fish (sardines, salmon – my personal favorite), especially cold-water fish since these contain the most omega-3s, is associated with a decreased risk of heart attack. They are loaded with DHA and EPA. They are very important for the formation of healthy brain and eye cells. If you don't feel like eating fish twice a week like I do, there is always fish oil.

Taken as a food supplement (I do, twice a day), fish oil is known to reduce triglycerides – an important risk factor for heart disease – from 10 to 33 percent, and even up to 40 percent in some research. Fish oil is also good for high blood pressure.

Another positive effect of fish oil is that it is anti-inflammatory. Scientists are more and more convinced that at least half of the heart diseases are caused by inflammation, even in people with "normal" cholesterol levels. My favorite fish oil is Barlean's Orange-flavored fish oil. You can also take Cod Liver oil (my mom used to give that to me. Yuk!) Now they make it flavorless, even flavored. Most recently, they came up with a child-friendly Smoothie Fish Oil but it contains sugar. You're better off "hiding" it in your kid's regular food.

- **Plant source**: Omega-3 fatty acids can also be found in seeds such as flaxseeds, chia seeds and some nuts like walnuts. In that case in the form of ALA (alphalinolenic acid) which is not as efficiently processed by our body. ALA to DHA and EPA will convert but with only about 20% efficiency. Although getting your omega-3s from plant source is a very good idea, especially if you're vegetarian, it will take more of it to be helpful to your health.

○ **The omega-6 fatty acids**, also called linoleic acids: Omega-6 fatty acids are converted to GLA (gamma linolenic acid) by our bodies if consumed directly from their natural source like raw pumpkin seeds, pine nuts, pistachio nuts, and sunflower seeds (and many other plant sources), Omega-6s are very beneficial to our health. Unfortunately, in our modern world, the vast majority of Omega-6s we ingest come from either refined oils (corn, peanut, safflower, soybean) processed with high heat and toxic chemicals (hexane), and/or from feedlot animals that are grain fed with corn. In a perfect world, the ratio of omega-6 to omega-3 in our diet should be from 1:1 to 3:1. Nowadays, the SAD (standard American diet) provides us an average of 15 times more omega-6s than omega-3s. If that was not bad enough, most of the industrialized omega-6s we consume are denatured (as in not natural) and oxidized by the manufacturing process. The high heat process, which is supposed to make these oils more shelf stable, turns their fatty acids from cis-fats (natural) to trans-fats (unnatural). You're probably already aware that Federal law has already banned trans-fatty acids in foods as they have been found to be much more detrimental to our health then even saturated fatty acids. These oxidized fats create inflammation in our body. A 2004 Time Magazine article titled " Inflammation: the Silent Killer" explains how modern degenerative diseases such as arthritis, high cholesterol and high blood pressure leading to atherosclerosis and heart attacks, Alzheimer disease, multiple sclerosis and even some forms of cancers are caused by inflammation. Feel free to check out the article.

Graisses et Huiles de Santé. *Healthy Fats and Oils*

Graisses et Huiles Saturées. *Saturated Fats and Oils.*

Raw or organic butter and Coconut oil.

Beurre de Ferme. *Farm Butter*

Even though my grandparents could not afford to keep a cow for milk and butter, we could find it daily at the local farmer's market. You need to know that my grandparents lived in the milk-producing region of France, Normandie, kind of like Wisconsin here. We could buy a mound of freshly churned deep yellow butter with a hint of sea salt (used as a natural preservative). It tasted almost like grass.

Why is raw fresh butter actually good for you?
Why do I suggest you eat raw or organic butter? Take a look at the long list of the benefits you receive when you include it in your diet:

1. Butter is rich in the most easily absorbable form of Vitamin A necessary for thyroid and adrenal health.
2. It contains lauric acid, important in treating fungal infections and candida.
3. It contains lecithin, essential for cholesterol metabolism.
4. It contains anti-oxidants that protect against free radical damage.
5. Food coming from grass fed cows contains CLA (conjugated linolenic acid), a healthy fat that has shown anticancer properties, is a muscle builder and boosts immunity.
6. It has anti-oxidants that protect against weakening arteries.
7. It is a great source of Vitamins E and K.
8. It is a very rich source of the vital mineral selenium.
9. Saturated fats in butter have strong anti-tumor and anti-cancer properties.
10. Vitamin D found in butter is essential to the absorption of calcium.
11. It protects against tooth decay.
12. It is your only source of an anti-stiffness factor (30% omega-3 fatty acids in grass-fed products), which protects against calcification of the joints.
13. Anti-stiffness factor in butter also prevents hardening of the arteries, cataracts, and calcification of the pineal gland.
14. It is a source of Activator X, which helps your body absorb minerals.

15. It is a source of iodine in a highly absorbable form.
16. It may promote fertility in women.
17. It is a source of quick energy, and is not stored in our bodies' adipose tissue.
18. The cholesterol found in butterfat is essential to children's brain and nervous system development.
19. It contains Arachidonic Acid (AA) which plays a role in brain function and is a vital component of cell membranes.
20. It protects against gastrointestinal infections in the very young and the elderly.

Why Raw or Organic Butter is Best
Believe me this is only a *partial* list. The best butter you can eat is raw or organic butter from a reputable dairy because pasteurization destroys nutrients. Unfortunately, the sale of raw butter is prohibited in most of our 50 states.

Alain's cooking tip
The good news is that, if you're willing, you can make your own butter. Buy organic heavy cream. Mix it with the same probiotic culture used to make yogurt. Let it sit at room temperature for 24 hours to allow for fermentation. Refrigerate overnight. Whisk it until it turns into butter. With a cheesecloth, drain the buttermilk (or save it for other uses) and voila! You have made your own homemade butter. It is called cultured butter. Here again, the secret is moderation. 1 to 2 pats of real butter a day will do you good.

Ghee
Another form of butter used for centuries in traditional Indian (Aryuvedic) cooking is Ghee or clarified butter. It has a lot of wonderful healing qualities. It is believed to strengthen the immune system and protect us from disease.

Huile Pure de Noix de Coco. *Pure or Virgin Coconut Oil*

For years, the oil industry has painted this healthy fat black. Why? I'm not sure. It might be due to the fact that when you look at the facts closely, you realize that coconut oil, even though it's a saturated fat, is a lot healthier for us than all the adulterated polyunsaturated oils that they peddle. Polyunsaturated oils are highly inflammatory once they have gone through their highly processed voyage, even though we are told they are healthy for you. Inflammation is what damages our arteries and cause heart disease. Marketing is king and negative advertising is particularly misleading in this case.

The coconut oil I'm referring to is not the hydrogenated fat used in some fast food restaurants. I'm talking about pure, virgin, unrefined, organic coconut oil. Unlike what we have been led to believe, the saturated fat in pure coconut oil has no adverse effects on cholesterol levels. In fact, researchers have found quite the opposite is true. If unrefined coconut oil was the cause of disease, then people living in countries like Sri Lanka, India and the Pacific Islands that use pure coconut oil in their daily diet would show evidence of heart diseases. In reality, these populations have very little heart disease.

A major study was performed in the 1960s on the remote islands of Pukapuka and Tokelau. The entire population of these islands was asked to take part in the study. Before the study, coconut oil, milk, and meat were the main staples in the diet contributing to 60% or more of the population's daily intake of calories from fat. Yet, these people showed no evidence of heart disease, high cholesterol, diabetes, cancer, or any other immunological or degenerative disease common in the Western World. In fact, they had never heard of heart disease or arthritis.

When researchers had half the population in the study begin eating a Western diet (refined and canned foods, sugars, polyunsaturated oils), they began to develop the diseases found in the Western world within days to weeks of adopting the new Western diet. When they returned to their traditional coconut-based diet, the diseases disappeared. Other interesting facts:

Coconut oil lowers LDL cholesterol. The cholesterol-lowering properties of coconut oil are a direct result of its ability to stimulate thyroid function. In the presence of adequate thyroid hormone, cholesterol (specifically LDL-cholesterol) is converted by enzymatic processes to the vitally necessary anti-aging steroids pregnenolone, progesterone and DHEA. These substances are required to help prevent heart disease, senility, obesity, cancer and other diseases associated with aging and chronic degenerative diseases.

Coconut oil stimulates thyroid function and is conducive to weight loss. Since coconut increases your thyroid's activity, it encourages weight loss. Polyunsaturated oils are known to decrease thyroid gland activity, thus lowering your metabolism and encouraging weight gain.

Coconut oil also has antiseptic properties. Unlike polyunsaturated oils, coconut oil does not oxidize (turn rancid) even after one year kept at room temperature. Coconut oil contains medium chain fatty acids (MCFAs) such as lauric, caprylic and myristic acids. Of these three, coconut oil contains 40% lauric acid, which has the greatest anti-viral activity of these three fatty acids. Lauric acid is so disease-fighting that it is present in breast milk.

Alain's shopping advice

The easiest way for you to find pure, virgin coconut oil is to go to the closest health food store. Spectrum and Barlean's are the best known brands. In Austin, you can find at Central Market and Whole Foods Market as well as many other stores. We even carry it at People's Pharmacy. Otherwise, look for it on the internet. There are plenty of good brands out there.

Alain's cooking tips

In the smoking point scale, coconut oil is higher than olive oil but lower than macadamia oil. So I use it for quick sautéing or omelets. For added flavor, I add a little butter to it. If you want to take advantage of its health benefits without cooking, feel free to add a teaspoon of it to your morning (or any time of the day) smoothie.

Graisses et Huiles Mono-insaturées. *Monounsaturated Fats and Oils*

Olive oil, Australian macadamia oil, avocado, almonds, cashews, peanuts, sesame seeds, pumpkin seeds and walnuts.

Monounsaturated fats possess a variety of key health benefits. Studies show that people who consume higher amounts of monounsaturated fats in their diets are healthier and thinner than their counterparts.

Monounsaturated fats are a unique type of fat found in particularly high quantities in olive oil. These stable fats decrease the oxidation of LDL cholesterol, help reduce cholesterol levels, and may partly explain why the "Mediterranean Diet", which is high in monounsaturated fats as well as whole foods, is protective against heart disease.

Assorted studies have revealed that populations that follow the "Mediterranean" diet, which is high in vegetables and whole grains, and low in saturated fats, but relatively high in total fat due to a high intake of olive oil, tend to have fairly low rates of cardiovascular disease and its associated mortality.

The Lyon's Mediterranean Diet study has shown that LDL cholesterol particles that contain monounsaturated fats, such as from olive oil, are much more resistant to oxidation that those that contain high levels of polyunsaturated fats, such as from other vegetable oils like corn or safflower oil. In addition, the substitution of monounsaturated fats for saturated fats in the diet has been shown to decrease total cholesterol by 13.4% and to decrease LDL cholesterol by 18%. The most important aspect of the use of monounsaturated fats is that they be used in place of saturated fats.

Huile de Graines de Chanvre. *Hemp Seed Oil*

Hemp seed oil contains an almost perfect mega-6 to omega-3 ratio of 3:1. It is not a widely produced oil because of hemp's other "qualities"; therefore it is imported from Canada, which has more stringent pesticide standards than the U.S. Even though it is imported, it is relatively easy to find in your favorite health food store in its organic, unrefined and cold-pressed state.

The majority of its omega-6 fatty acid is GLA (gamma linolenic acid), the "good" omega-6 found in evening primrose and borage oils. The famous Harvard Nurses' Health Study proves that the good omega-6 fatty acids lower LDL (bad) cholesterol.

Alain's shopping advice

Since it is still fairly hard to find, most likely you will only be able to find in health food stores or on the internet. In Austin, I have found it at both Whole Foods and Central Market.

Alain's cooking tips

As the omega-3 fatty acids contained in this oil are heat sensitive, I would only recommend it for salad dressing or as a drizzle on top of steamed vegetables. Keep it in your refrigerator when you are not using it.

Huile de Noix de Macadamia. *Macadamia Nut Oil*

Macadamia Nut Oil is also one of the highest oil in monounsaturated fats. It has an even richer content of monounsaturated oil than olive oil. How about that! It is composed of approximately 85 percent of it, including the heart-friendly oleic acid. The combination of oleic acid and omega-3 fatty acids contained in this oil lower triglycerides and improve HDL (good) cholesterol levels. This is exactly what we're trying to accomplish.

Macadamia Nut Oil has the ideal ratio of omega-3 to omega-6 fatty acids. That is, 1:1 or equal amounts of each. That ratio is the healthiest ratio for our body's health. Nowadays, because of the large amount of processed vegetable oils available, we are ingesting a large amount of mega-6 fatty acids, which are inflammatory. Ideally, to become healthier, you need to balance your omega-6 to omega-3 ratio as close as possible to 1:1. Macadamia nut oil offers you a near perfect omega balance.

Alain's shopping advice

It has a buttery taste, a golden, yellow color and high amounts of naturally occurring anti-oxidants. Try to buy cold-pressed macadamia nut oil. My favorite brand is MacNutOil from Australia.

Alain's cooking tips

On the cooking side of business, macadamia oil has a much higher smoking point – 410F - (the temperature at which an overheated oil becomes oxidized and toxic to our body) than all monounsaturated oils. You can use macadamia nut oil to cook, sauté, bake, and stir-fry. There is less danger of creating the toxic trans-fatty acids and free radicals when this oil is heated to high temperatures. If you can afford it, use macadamia oil for pan-frying, but still be careful not to overheat it.

Huile d'Olive. *Olive oil*

Olives and olive oil are the staples of Mediterranean cuisine. It also is a monounsaturated fat, which is a type of fat known to lower LDL (bad) cholesterol and raise the heart-friendly HDL (good) cholesterol. Even though olive oil is a relatively stable fat, it is important not to use olive oil when cooking foods at high temperatures. Exposing even this stable oil to high temperatures will cause it to oxidize and become damaging to your health.

What makes olive oil so healthy for us: Polyphenols

The Polyphenols in olive oil are primarily responsible for its cardiovascular benefits.

Polyphenols are known to have anti-inflammatory, antioxidant and anticoagulant properties. Evidence is growing that olive oil may protect against colon cancer and osteoporosis. The purer the olive oil is, the more polyphenols it contains.

Alain's shopping advice

I always buy cold-pressed extra virgin olive oil. Extra virgin means that it is the least processed form of oil. It comes out of the first pressing. Make sure it's cold-pressed, as heat will destroy all of its essential fatty acids, vitamins and antioxidant benefits. Since I prefer a lighter flavor, I tend to pick olive oil that comes from Italy, as olive oil coming from Spain tends to have a stronger flavor. In Austin, I find that the organic extra virgin oil offered at Central Market is a very good product at a reasonable price. Nowadays, it is a lot easier to find olive oil, so your neighborhood grocery should carry a few good quality brands. Oops! I almost forgot. Always store your extra virgin olive oil in an opaque or dark bottle or better yet, in a metal container. You see, since light is oxidative to fresh oil, it will turn your golden oil into rancid oil. At home, keep it in the dark at room temperature if you plan to use it fairly quickly, or in the refrigerator. If is of good quality, it will congeal in the cold. Not to worry, just run it under warm water for a while and it will be ready to use.

Alain's cooking tips

When heating olive oil, sprinkle a little water into it, just a few drops. When the water "sings", your oil is hot enough to cook.

Alain's Recipes: *Alain's Healing Salad Dressing, page 251. Avocado Sauce, page 253. Lemon Cream Sauce, page 254.*

Fibres. *Fiber*

Fiber - particularly *soluble* fiber - can lower cholesterol levels and may help you to lose weight as well. Since it takes more time to chew high fiber foods, it allows your body to feel full faster and for a longer period. The result is that you're less likely to overeat. Examples of high fiber foods are bran, oatmeal, beans, the vast majority of green vegetables, and fruits like raspberries, raisins, avocados (yes, it's a fruit), as well as the fruits for old folks: prunes. Here are a few high fiber foods:

Céréales. *Grains*

Some doctors in our alternative medicine community consider all grains to be a danger to human health. In their opinion, the vast majority of over-processed modern grains do not compare favorably to the ancient grains our ancestors used to pick and grind for their rustic flat breads. Not to mention the new genetically engineered Frankenfoods that scare the "Petit Jesus" out of me!

I'm not as strict as some of my colleagues. Besides, could I even pretend to be French without eating a little French baguette once in a while? And, unlike a lot of my private clients, I am not gluten-sensitive nor do I have Celiac disease. That does not mean I cannot help people with these conditions; I do. But if you are not adversely affected by gluten, a little grain once in a while can be a good thing. As always, use moderation and do not scarf down that French baguette whole in one sitting.

Here are a few grains that can actually help lower your cholesterol.

Flocons d'Avoine. *Oatmeal*

You knew that one was coming! Oatmeal is accepted by all sides of the nutritional debate as a potentially beneficial cereal. For one thing, it's loaded with both kinds of fiber: soluble and insoluble. Soluble fiber feeds your friendly bacteria and insoluble acts as a colon scrubber. Oatmeal contains 55 percent soluble and 45 percent insoluble fiber: a good balance.

The beta-glucans contained in the soluble fiber are what boost your immune system. Beta-glucans are a kind of polysaccharide (a form of long-chain saccharides or glucose molecule) that helps lower your cholesterol and triglycerides levels and significantly reduces the possibility of cardiovascular disease and stroke. One bowl of oatmeal eaten at breakfast every day can reduce your total cholesterol from 8 to 23 percent.

A serving (1/3 cup for me) contains 5 g of fiber. Oatmeal also contains the largest amount of protein of any popular breakfast cereal. One cup of oatmeal contains 4 g of protein per 1/3 cup. But, beware, gluten-sensitive or Celiac sufferers out there, this is the kind of protein that will make you sick. Stay away! For all others, enjoy oatmeal's health benefits without guilt.

Alain's shopping advice

From the healthiest to the least desirable: groats are oatmeal without the hull, the closest to its natural state. But they're kind of hard to find unless you're lucky to have a health food store like Whole Foods Market in your neighborhood (I'm still waiting for their endorsement check. Just kidding!). They require the longest cooking time, about 20 minutes. Easier to find and still very good for you are steel-cut oats, also known as Irish or Scottish oats, which need less cooking time but provide the same health kick. Rolled oats are also acceptable as long as they are the old-fashioned kind and thick. Bulk and organic are your best choice.

Alain's cooking tips

In America, it is customary to cook your oatmeal. Not true everywhere. I get mine in the form of unsweetened Swiss Muesli which does not require cooking.

Alain's Recipes: *A Votre Santé Healthy Breakfast, page 172.*

Riz Complet. *Brown Rice*

Now, don't be confused, I'm not talking of the Uncle You Know Who kind of rice. That refined type of rice is useless for human consumption (and I mean that in a nice way). It has very little nutritional value, and it pushes your blood sugar level through the roof, which eventually leads to high triglycerides levels. Avoid it if you want to stay healthy. On the other hand, the unrefined version is loaded with good nutrition. For one thing, it still has the bran on it, which is fiber. Since brown rice only has the outer hull removed, it still contains nutrients such as niacin (which is a vitamin known to reduce cholesterol), vitamin B6, magnesium, manganese, selenium and vitamin E.

A cup of cooked brown rice possesses 4 g of mostly insoluble fiber, known for protecting you from an assortment of cancers like colon, breast and prostate. But for us, high-cholesterol folks, you'll be glad to learn that its fiber and phytonutrients content help lower cholesterol levels and prevent cardiovascular diseases. *Aryzanol*, a type of rice oil (italics) helps lower cholesterol as well. The Camargue region of Southern France (to the West of Marseille) is well known for growing rice for most of Europe. I have a few native recipes for you.

Alain's shopping advice

In France, I would naturally choose brown rice from Camargue, but since it's not available here, this is what I do: I buy organic brown rice at the bulk section. Buying bulk is better for your pocketbook because it's cheaper (you don't have to pay for additional packaging) and for the environment (minimal throw away packaging). Typically, when you buy from a store with high volume, buying bulk will provide you with a fresher product. Some stores (not many, I know) will actually allow you to bring your own recycled container.

Alain's cooking tips

If you want stickier rice, buy short grain rice. If your dish requires a non-sticky rice, use medium-long or long grain rice. For my own part, I mostly use rice in my **Easy Tomato, Rice and Beans** recipe.

Alain's Recipes: *Salad from the Camargue Region, page 242. Alain's Easy Tomato, Rice and Beans Recipe, page 199.*

Haricots Secs et Légumineuses. *Beans and Légumes*

Haricots Secs. *Dried Beans*

Beans have both positive and negative qualities; however, the good far outweighs the bad. On the negative side, beans contain a substance call *lectin*.

According to Loren Cordain, Ph.D., author of the world-renowned book "The Paleo Diet" and a highly respected researcher at the University of Colorado, beans, legumes, grains, seeds and yeast may be blamed for a series of autoimmune diseases in genetically sensitive people. The lectin protein may be the culprit here. It is suspected to cause intestinal permeability (also called leaky gut syndrome), which allows some food proteins to pass through the intestinal wall and create food allergies.

On the beneficial side, beans are loaded with fiber. As a matter of fact, it is one of the best sources of fiber in the plant world. The truth is, most of us do not get enough fiber from our diet. The fiber contained in beans and legumes are now known to lower cholesterol, improve our intestinal health and protect us from an assortment of degenerative diseases such as cancer, heart disease, diabetes and obesity. In the old, pre-industrial days, our ancestors used to get an average of 50 to 100 grams of fiber a day. What do you think is our average daily intake of fiber these days? 11 grams. Institutions such as the National Cancer Institute and the U.S. Dietary Guidelines recommend we get at least 25 grams of fiber a day. It is even recommended that we increase that to 30-35 grams. Can we do that? Yes, if we pay attention to what we eat. I will provide you with recipes containing plenty of fiber.

For example, a cup of beans such as kidney beans will provide us with 11 g of fiber. Even better, the same amount of adzuki beans (black Japanese beans) will give us up to 17 g of fiber per serving. According to the Nutrition Department at the University of Kentucky, a cup of cooked beans a day can lower your total cholesterol by 10 percent in as little as 6 weeks. A study conducted by that same university showed that eating ½ cup of navy and pinto beans a day for 3 weeks lowered the cholesterol level of these subjects by an amazing 19 percent. I know, who wants to eat a cup of beans every day unless it's part of your culture? Don't worry; I give you plenty of variety of choices to get fiber in your diet.

As an additional benefit, most of the beans are loaded with antioxidants. As I mentioned before, oxidation or inflammation of your arteries are believed to be the main cause for plaque buildup. So antioxidants are very important. Red beans, red kidney beans and pinto beans are ranked by the USDA antioxidant ranking as some of the highest antioxidant ratings of any foods. For heart health, folic acid is a very important factor. Some beans such as adzuki beans, black-eyed peas, lentils and pinto beans are loaded with it. And to top it off, beans are loaded with magnesium, iron, zinc and potassium, and molybdenum, a trace mineral known to improve the beneficial qualities of digestive enzymes. Typically, a cup of beans contains an average of 15 g of fiber as well as being a good source of plant-based protein. Beans also contain complex carbohydrates, digest slowly and do not affect your blood sugar level.

The French flageolets (also called "chevrier" as they used to be eaten by "les chevres", goats) are a type of white bean grown in the region of Arpajon that is harvested before full maturity and dried while still green. This makes them very tender, buttery and flavorful. In the Southern Alps, they are usually served with lamb as a traditional meal for Easter, but can be enjoyed any time. They are very special to my heart as they bring back fond memories of Easter meals shared with my family.

Alain's shopping advice

I buy my dried beans in bulk and organic. If cooking beans from scratch is a time challenge, buy quality organic canned or jarred beans. As they need a long cooking time either way, you might as well let the manufacturer do it for you. And the good news is that there is no noticeable nutritional difference between the two.

Alain's cooking tips

Before soaking your beans, spread them on a light-colored plate and pick out any stones or debris. To avoid the potentially socially embarrassing side effect of eating beans, make sure to soak them overnight in cold filtered water, or, if you forgot to do that, try this alternative method: Boil your beans for 2 minutes, cover and let soak for at least two hours. Make sure to get rid of the soaking water and rinse your beans well before cooking. I typically use twice the amount of filtered water as beans. Another trick is, if you want your beans to be tender, never salt them before cooking. It will make them tougher and you will need a much longer time to cook them. Use three cups of water per cup of dried beans.

There are two ways to cook beans. Place your rinsed beans in a regular cast iron pot. Using a 3 to 1 ratio, make sure the beans are covered by 1 inch of water. Bring them to boil, cover with a lid, lower the heat to medium-low and simmer for up to an hour and a half.

The other method is my favorite: the pressure cooker. Using only 2 cups of water per cup of beans, I bring them to a boil, close the lid, allow the pressure to build until the lid is tightly sealed, lower the heat to medium-low (just make sure to maintain the pressure) and cook for 30 minutes. When the time is up, set the cooker aside and let cool naturally until the pressure indicator is down. If you're in a hurry you can run cold water over the closed lid of the cooker to help the pressure come down. Be careful to follow the instructions given by the manufacturer. Pressure-cooking nowadays is a very safe, quick and economical way to cook. Both my grandmother and my mother used pressure cookers and cooked good meals with them.

Alain's Recipes: *Fresh Fava Bean Soup, page194. Pesto Soup page 190. Spring Vegetable Minestrone, page 192. Alain's Easy Tomato, Rice and Beans Recipe, page 199. Green Flageolets with Thyme and Pine Nuts, page 200.*

Pois Chiches. *Garbanzo Beans or Chickpeas*

Garbanzo beans, as well as other beans, lentils and peas are part of a family of food called legumes or pulses. The amount of fiber (12.5 g per cup) in these beans help lower blood cholesterol and slows the absorption of sugars, which is also very important for people with diabetes. Another benefit a lot of people are not aware of is that eating foods like beans forces us to take the time to chew our food, which slows down the digestive process and allows us to feel fuller faster and helps us avoid overstuffing ourselves. You see, our bodies have a natural way to give us a "Stop!" signal when we have eaten enough. It's called satiety, a fancy word for feeling full. The problem is, it takes a little time for that signal to light up. In these days of fast food and faster eating, we do not allow enough time for our body to give us that signal and we tend to overeat. When eaten slowly, fiber will fill us up and help us lose weight. But for that to happen, we must take the time necessary to allow your body to do its job and let us know we've had enough.

Chickpeas contain a perfect 1:1 ratio of calcium and magnesium, a nice amount of folate and a good dose of heart-healthy potassium (477 mg per cup). An additional benefit is that they contain the powerful antioxidant selenium and provide us with 2 ounces of vegetable protein per serving.

Alain's shopping advice

Although purists would have you cook your garbanzo beans from scratch, it is much easier and faster to use a quality organic canned variety.

Alain's cooking tips

For dried garbanzo beans, use the same tips offered in the beans paragraph. Otherwise, use a good quality can opener and be careful not to cut your self on the sharp edge of the opened lid. I should know, it happened to me quite a few times. Actually, I'm more afraid of can lids than my favorite chef's knife!

<u>Alain's Recipes</u>: *Peoples Pharmacy Hummus, page 178.*

Lentilles. *Lentils*

Lentils have been part of the Mesopotamian and Middle Eastern cultures for millenniums. Do you remember the old story in Genesis of Esau giving up his birthright to Jacob for a meal of lentils? What most people don't know is that they also lower cholesterol. Lentils can be brown, green or red. The brown in the most commonly used, the green are mostly grown and used in France, and the red are used and eaten mainly in the Middle East and India.

Lentils are a traditional source of protein for vegetarian cultures and contain 18 g per cup. It also contains 16 g of fiber, primarily soluble fiber, which helps trap excess cholesterol and escort it out of our bodies. Lentils also provide a good amount of folate, as well as iron and manganese.

Alain's shopping advice

Again, I would suggest you buy your lentils from the bulk section. Organic is best. Store them in a dry, cool place, if possible away from the light.

Alain's cooking tips

Unlike beans, lentils do not need to be soaked. They can be cooked right away. Use 3 cups of water for 1 cup of lentils. Bring your water to boil. I learned a long time ago from one of my chefs that placing lentils in boiling water will make them more digestible. Before you rinse them, spread the amount of lentils you need on a light-colored plate and pick out any stones. No matter how long you cook them, the stones will never get tender! Place your lentils in a strainer and rinse them thoroughly. When the water is boiling, add the lentils into the boiling water carefully. Green lentils take about 30 minutes to cook, red lentils about 20 minutes. If you prefer them a little more firm or need them for a salad, cook them 5 minutes less.

Alain's Recipes: *Lentil Tomato Soup with Spinach, page 186. Traditional Du Puy Lentil Soup, page 188. Lentils Salad with Bacon and Dried Ham, page 248.*

Légumes. *Vegetables*

Alain's General Vegetable Shopping Advice

Unless otherwise specified, this is how I would suggest you buy your vegetables: the freshest picked, with the least impact on the environment.

1. Shop locally and in season. If you have access to it, buy from your local farmer's market, farmer's co-op, or directly from the farm. Get to know your local farmers. Some of them even offer weekly or monthly baskets where you receive an assortment of vegetables and fruits in season for a certain price. Eating food harvested in season from the area in which you live is the best way of ensuring that your food is at the peak of its freshness. It also supports your local economy and avoids hurting the environment through long-range shipping. Typically, local farmers are too small to be able to afford Certified Organic Certification. To make sure they're not unloading produce from somewhere else in their own crates, talk to them at the market. Ask to visit their farm, take a tour and ask a lot of questions. Local farmers are proud of the products they sell you and will be happy to show you around their farm. In Austin, our best-known local farm is **Boggy Creek Farm**, but there are plenty of other high quality farms nearby. Use Google to find local farmers markets or farmers advertising their fresh wares. In Austin, there's a new way to get your local and organic foods from local farmers without having to go to the markets: **Greenling** (greenling.com). You can order online or by phone and they will deliver to your door for a reasonable fee. If your time is very precious, this is a great way to eat healthy food without running around all over the place.

2. While in your favorite grocery store, buy produce from farmers located in your state. It's not quite as good, but the next best solution. If possible, buy organic products or ask your produce person for advice.

3. In your grocery store, look for organic produce shipped from other states, the closer to your state, the better. Every mile counts.

4. Another good solution is to buy flash-frozen organic vegetables. They are frozen as soon as they are picked and keep most of their nutrients in the process. Only defrost what you will use. To prevent freezer burn, use

containers with tight-fitting lids to store the unused portion. Do not refreeze defrosted vegetables.

5. Bar all of the above, buy produce only in season and wash it carefully in cold water with a few drops of organic soap or a special produce-washing solution. This may be the only way you can access fresh produce. Better not-so-perfect produce than no produce at all!

6. If possible, avoid buying from countries that may not have the same health and environmental laws we have in the United States. Their laws may be more relaxed than ours and your produce may be covered with pesticides that are banned here.

Artichauts. *Artichokes*

Artichokes contain a nice amount of silymarin, an ingredient known to cleanse the liver. Also, the standardized extract has been tested as a treatment for high cholesterol and triglycerides. In laboratory, the flavonoids extracted from artichokes, especially *luteolin* have prevented the oxidation of LDL ("bad") cholesterol, a confirmed risk factor for cardiovascular disease.

Do you remember the fiber we talked about earlier? One large artichoke contains up to 9 g of fiber for a measly 60 calories. The best of both worlds: high fiber and low calories. It also contains about 72 mg of the marvelous magnesium, 425 mg of potassium, a little bit of folate and the eye-friendly lutein and zeaxanthin.

Alain's shopping advice

Artichokes can range in size from baby artichokes of 2 to 3 ounces each, to jumbo artichokes. In my opinion, the smaller, the better. Artichokes should be firm, compact, and heavy for their size, and have an even green color in the spring and summer. While nobody is watching, give them a squeeze, and if they squeak, you know they are fresh.

Artichokes dehydrate rapidly, so as soon as you get home, put them in a plastic bag and sprinkle a little water inside the bag (not too much or your artichokes will get moldy) and store it in the vegetable bin of the refrigerator.

Alain's cooking tips

Typically, not a lot of people like to eat artichokes because they require a lot of work to get to the "heart" of the matter. So they eat canned artichoke hearts, which is not a bad thing, but canned artichokes do not even begin to taste like fresh ones. But there are two ways to get around that problem. Do it the French way: steam them for 10-12 minutes. Let them cool down a bit while preparing a nice dipping vinaigrette made of red wine vinegar, sea salt, freshly ground black pepper, Dijon mustard and olive oil whisked together (see vinaigrette recipe). Others prefer to dip them in a freshly done mayonnaise. Then you grab the whole artichoke, peel each leaf one at a time and dip the fleshy part in the vinaigrette or mayonnaise, scrape the flesh with your front teeth and pile the used leaves on a separate plate. Keep on doing that until you reach the heart. Remove the "foin" ("hairs") as we call them in France, keeping the heart. Cut it up in pieces; toss it in the remaining vinaigrette and savor. Miam! (Yum!). That's the way we eat them in my family. Now, I realize that's not exactly fast food but that's the way they should be enjoyed. One slow bite at a time, savoring the experience with friends or family, with a glass of cool Vin de Provence.

The other way is to enjoy them as "Artichauts a la Barigoule" or Artichokes Barigoule, the way they are traditionally cooked in the South of France. When I used to work at the Moulin de Mougins near Cannes, Chef Roger Verge used to make his own world-famous version. See my version in the recipe section.

If you want the goodness without the hard work, use good quality canned artichoke hearts, drain and slice them to add to your favorite mixed green salad.

Alain's Recipes: *Artichoke Hearts a la Barigoule, page 202.*

Topinambours. *Jerusalem Artichokes*

They are also called "poires de terre" (earth pears) in contrast to "pommes de terre" (earth apples also known as potatoes). To this day, I still remember my grandmother (Mamie) telling how, during World War II, while escaping the Germans, they had to steal topinambours out of the fields along their escape route and eat them raw. Obviously they survived that ordeal but I wouldn't have liked to be in their place. Traditionally, topinambours were grown to feed "les cochons" (pigs).

Don't get fooled by the name, these wonderful roots are not really artichokes. And they're not even from Jerusalem. Someone played a joke on us when naming this vegetable. They are members of the sunflower family and are sometimes called *sunchokes*. If you're not sure what they look like, they resemble a rounder version of ginger root but with a mild flavor. They make a wonderful and lower-calorie version of baked potatoes. They can also be shredded raw and added to your salad. It's a good idea to sprinkle them with freshly squeezed lemon juice to prevent them from oxidizing and turning brown.

What makes this vegetable worth eating is its surprisingly large amount of *fructooligosaccharides* and *inulin*. What are those? They are happy foods for your intestinal flora. In my opinion and that of many nutritionists, our immune system health starts in our gut. If you keep your "good" bacteria happy and well fed, they will help you digest your food and fend off the "bad" bacteria and viruses.

So, ideally, your acidophilus and bifidus (friendly bacteria) would love to at fructooligosaccharides and inulin for breakfast, lunch and dinner. They are called "prebiotics" - health food - for your "probiotics" - good bacteria. And inulin is a form of soluble fiber that was found to lower blood glucose, LDL cholesterol and triglycerides as well as inhibit the growth of an assortment of cancers in a study published in *The Journal of Nutrition*. Inulin can also be found in asparagus and dandelion.

Gas alert!!! Some people are sensitive to inulin and may feel intestinal inconvenience, otherwise known as flatulence. You have been warned!

Alain's shopping advice

To make your life easier, try to pick Jerusalem Artichokes that are even in size. They should be firm, plump and have an obvious fresh appearance. Avoid Jerusalem Artichokes exhibiting a greenish color, wrinkles, blotches, or signs of sprouting. Bumps and unevenness on the skin are just fine. Store them in a plastic bag in the refrigerator's vegetable bin. They will last about a week, but I recommend you use them right away.

Alain's cooking tips

Don't forget that sunchokes are root vegetables so get that veggie brush out and use some elbow grease to get the dirt off. (In France, we use the term "huile de coude" or elbow oil. Why do the Americans use grease and French oil? Maybe that's the reason the French are healthier!) Make sure not to scrub the skin away. It is full of vitamins and minerals.

Jerusalem artichokes are extremely versatile, and can be cooked or used raw. You can cut them coarsely and steam them for 5-7 minutes, then add your favorite dressing and savor them. You can also dice or shred them and cook them quickly in a stir-fry dish, surrounded by other assorted vegetables and a little extra virgin olive oil. Jerusalem Artichokes are also wonderful sautéed, baked or boiled, and seasoned as you might season a baked potato. When raw, they are a crisp and crunchy like jicama, and can be added to a variety of salads and slaws. Another idea is to use them with your favorite dip. Since they tend to oxidize and turn brown quickly, I would suggest you prepare them just before you eat them. If that is not possible, you can also soak them in water with lemon juice.

Alain's Recipes: *Braised Garlic Roasted Jerusalem Artichokes, page 203.*

Ail. *Garlic*

Garlic's culinary and medicinal attributes have been known since ancient times. The oldest mention of garlic was as far back as the time that the Giza pyramids were built. The Greeks and Romans were very fond of it as a medicine as well. Have you ever tried pasta sauce without garlic? In France we would say: "c'est comme un baiser sans moustache" (it's like a kiss without the mustache). The largest garlic producer in the world is China, but I still much prefer the small, fragrant garlic grown in the South of France.

Garlic, as well as shallots, chives, leeks and onions, is part of the allium family. *Allicin,* one of garlic compounds released when a garlic clove is crushed or chopped, has a known anti-platelet effect. That is, it prevents platelets in our blood from sticking together (coagulating) and is known as a blood thinner. Garlic in more than 1,200 studies has proven to be LDL-lowering, antihypersensitive (anti-high blood pressure), antioxidant (counter the negative effects of free radicals), antimicrobial (kills microbes) and antiparasitic (kills the bugs).

German researchers found that subjects taking nearly one gram of garlic per day (900 mg) had up to an 82% reduction in the plaque volume in their arteries, compared to controls who took a "dummy" placebo powder instead. Garlic is believed to work by making blood less "sticky," preventing the clinging of plaque to arterial walls. These results substantiate that garlic may have more than a preventive effect and even possibly, in the researchers' words, "a curative role in arteriosclerosis therapy (plaque regression)." In other words, garlic can help reduce plaque. Not bad for one little bulb!

In a meta-analysis conducted in England, after 4 weeks of testing, garlic supplements were found to lower total cholesterol by 12 percent. It also lowered LDL (bad) cholesterol from 5 to 15 percent while at the same time raise HDL (good) cholesterol by up to 22 percent. Not only that, it also lowered triglycerides levels by 17 percent. One of the major causes of high triglycerides is the ingestion of excess sugar and sweeteners. Triglycerides are created when the glucose that is not needed by your body is transformed into fat and lodges around your waist and hips. It is a component of LDL (bad) cholesterol and increasingly, scientists are regarding high triglycerides levels as potentially more dangerous than total cholesterol levels.

Alain's shopping advice

If at all possible try to find locally grown garlic. It will always be fresher and a little stronger than the type coming from China. Pick nicely shaped garlic heads, with no dried out or moldy cloves.

Alain's cooking tips

Honesty, being from La Cote d'Azur, I like mine raw, especially in salad dressing (vinaigrette) and mayonnaise, especially "Aïoli", a mayonnaise loaded with raw garlic that we French use with white fish, cold meat and cooked potatoes. If you are not used to preparing mayonnaise from scratch, you can buy good quality mayonnaise in a jar (Spectrum) and add crushed garlic cloves to it. It is also used liberally in the mayonnaise-like sauce called "Rouille", which means rusty in French. This sauce is used only for the famous "soupe de poisson" (fish soup), of which you will find hundreds of variations in the South of France. The two are inseparable. The proper way to eat "soupe de poisons" is to spread the "rouille" on top of toasted French baguette rounds, drop it in the soup and eat it all with a good spoonful of soup. Miam! (Yum!).

I also use it in my healing green soup. When I feel a cold or flu coming, I prepare this simple but special soup, drink two bowls of it, go to bed and sweat it out. Usually I'm fine in the morning.

Alain's Recipes: *Small Onion Tarts with Niçoises Black Olives, page 180. Alain's Healthy Green Soup, page 182. Red Wine Onion Soup, page 184. Provencal Sage and Garlic Soup, page 187. Aïoli sauce, page 252.*

Poireau. *Leeks*

It still amazes me that leeks are still under-appreciated in the US when they are so popular in France. Think of them as a sweeter version of onions. Leeks are card-carrying members of the allium family like onions, garlic, green onions and shallots. Increased consumption of this family of vegetables is linked to lower cases of prostate and colon cancers. But more to the point for us, they also lower levels of LDL ("bad") cholesterol and can lower blood pressure.

One low calorie (54) leek also provides a good amount of eye-healthy lutein and zeaxanthin, carotenoids known for their ability to prevent macular degeneration, unfortunately the number one cause of blindness in elderly folks. Leeks also contain a good amount of fiber (here's that fiber again), more than 1,400 IUS of vitamin A, calcium, iron, magnesium, phosphorus, potassium and vitamin K, a vitamin important for blood clotting.

Alain's shopping advice

I like my leeks to be firm and straight with dark green leaves and white necks. Do not pick leeks that are yellowed or wilted. Make sure the bulb is not cracked or bruised. I prefer to purchase small, tender leeks. Now that leeks are better known, they are available year round. Ideally, get them from your local farmer. They will be glad for the business and you will have a very fresh leek.

You should store your leeks unwashed and untrimmed in the vegetable section of your refrigerator, where they will keep fresh for a week or two. To keep them moist, keep them wrapped in the plastic bag they came in.

Alain's cooking tips

I like them steamed for 6-8 minutes (depending on size) and drizzled with extra virgin olive oil, lemon juice, and a crush of sea salt and black pepper. That's the way it is usually served in French health spas. If this form does not appeal to you, try my version of the famous Vichyssoise Soup or mix them in your stir-fried vegetables. Caution: Cooked leeks are highly perishable, and even when kept in the refrigerator, will only stay fresh for about two days. Eat them while still warm from the steamer. That's when they're the best.

Alain's Recipes: *Butternut Squash Vichyssoise Soup, page 196.*

Champignons. *Mushrooms*

Mushrooms have been used for centuries in Eastern medicine. Why not in Western cultures? It's a mystery to me. Although I do not specialize in Eastern medicine, I know how to prepare them, eat them and I know they're good for you. In a way, it makes sense. Mushrooms are a large form of fungus and usually grow on decaying matter. In France the famous Champignon de Paris are grown in caves on horse manure (mais oui!)

The most famous medicinal mushrooms are Maitake, Shiitake and Reishi mushrooms. They are mostly know for their anti-cancer properties but in Japanese studies, consumption of shiitake mushrooms has been shown to lower blood cholesterol by as much as 45 percent due to an active compound called *eritadenine*. Closer to home, the Crimini mushrooms and even the Champignons de Paris (white button mushrooms) are replete with nutrients.

Alain's shopping advice

Most stores nowadays will allow you to pick your own mushrooms. That's the way it should be. Mushrooms should be firm, plump and clean. Do not pick those that are wrinkled or have wet slimy spots. Mushrooms tend to darken as they age, so pick those that are either creamy white (for button mushrooms) or tan (for Crimini mushrooms). If your recipe calls for caps only, choose mushrooms that have short stems to avoid waste. A wide variety of mushrooms is available throughout the year, even the exotic types.

The best way to store mushrooms is to keep them in the refrigerator on any shelf, not in the vegetable bin. That is too humid for them and will turn them soggy. Instead, place them in a paper bag and either wrap that bag in a wet towel or in a plastic bag to prevent them from drying out. Dried mushrooms should be stored in a tightly sealed container in either the refrigerator or freezer, where they will stay fresh for six months to one year.

Alain's cooking tips

To clean them of possible dirt, use a barely wet towel and wipe them gently. Do not soak them in water as they are like little sponges and will get soggy on you. If you use them with the stem, trim the bottom of the stem before you cook them. If you need only the buttons (chapeau), gently break off the stem and save it for a vegetable soup or to make a vegetable broth.

Alain's Recipes: *Ham-stuffed Portobello Mushrooms, page 205. Gnocchis with Mushroom Sauce, page 206.*

Poivrons Épicés. *Hot Peppers: Cayenne, Chile, Jalapeno, Poblano*

You may be surprised but one study showed that capsaicin, the active ingredient in hot peppers, may help lower LDL cholesterol. This may need further research but it's good news for Texans, who love to dip their tortilla chips in fiery salsa. I'll be honest with you: we don't use a lot of hot peppers in the South of France but if you'll allow me, I'll sneak in a couple of non-French recipes from my adopted state, Texas.

Alain's shopping advices

The best peppers have vivid, deep colors and glossy, firm and taut skins. Their stems should seem hardy and fresh. Avoid those that are wrinkled or have soft areas or black spots. They should not have any cracks near the stem end.

You should store your unwashed peppers in paper bags or wrap in paper towels and store them in the vegetable compartment of your refrigerator. They should last for at least one week. Do not store peppers in plastic bags as this will likely result in moisture accumulation, which will cause them to spoil.

Alain's cooking tips

Don't make the mistake I once did: I was working with hot peppers with my bare hands and wiped my eyes. Do you think I learned a lesson then? Not even a girl made me cry like that before. Since then, I wear rubber gloves while chopping hot peppers. And just to be sure, wash your knife and cutting board thoroughly after cutting your peppers.

The stinging component, capsaicin, is primarily found in the seeds and fleshy white inner membranes. If you want to enjoy the pungency of peppers but minimize their heat, you can remove these parts, although capsaicin is responsible for much of chili peppers' healing properties.

Please remember that there is a range of "hotness" between pepper varieties and sometimes also within the same variety. You may need to adjust the amount you use each time you cook with them, even if they are the same type. If you're bold enough, taste a little piece of pepper before adding it to your recipe to determine the level of heat, so you will know how much to add.

Alain's Recipes: *As much as I'd like to, nothing beats a good Texan salsa, not even a French one so I won't insult your intelligence.*

Petit Pois Verts (Green Peas)

When I was a kid, green peas were one of the few "green" vegetables I loved to eat. What I did not know was that my mother was adding a little sugar in the cooking water to make them more palatable. I also loved to play around with my peas and make funny faces with them in my mashed potatoes.

Peas are a good source of fiber (5.5 g in fresh, 8 g in dried split peas per ½ cup serving). They contain a good amount of vitamin A, vitamin K and 5 g of plant-based protein per serving.

You can use them fresh, flash frozen or dried in an assortment of yummy dishes provided here.

Alain's shopping advice

That's a tough one. I have to admit that since I left my Mamie's farm, I haven't had a chance to liberate peas from their pods. Who's got the time anyway? That was fine when I was a little kid and had nothing better to do (besides, I didn't have the choice, if you know what I mean) but as a busy adult, I don't do it anymore. So I cheat. I buy my green peas (also called garden peas) frozen and organic. They're re picked and shelled at the peak of freshness and flash frozen. That's good enough for me.

Alain's cooking tips

I like to steam them with sliced young carrots, and then toss them while they're still hot with a pat of fresh butter, sea salt and black pepper. Sometimes, simple is best. You get all the freshness, flavor and goodness that way. Of course, I love them in soups and "jardinière de legumes" (assortment of fresh vegetables).

<u>Alain's Recipes</u>: *Green Pea Soup with Mint, page 181.*

Autres Légumes. *Other Vegetables*

Obviously, all vegetables are good for you. We should all eat a variety of them. They all contain soluble and non-soluble fiber, able to help lower your bad cholesterol levels and increase your good cholesterol levels. They are all loaded with antioxidants that will prevent cholesterol oxidation and prevent plaque creation and deposit in your arteries. I cannot possibly list all known vegetables here; I chose to write about the vegetables known to lower your cholesterol. But that should not stop you from eating a wide assortment of beautiful fresh, colorful vegetables in season.

Other vegetables wonderful for your health are: Arugula, Asparagus, Beets, Bok Choy, Broccoli, Broccoli Rabe, Brussels sprouts (my personal favorite), Cabbage, Carrots, Cauliflower, Celery, Collard greens, Dandelion, Eggplant, Endive, Fennel, Green Beans and Haricots Verts (a French, smaller, stringless, more tender version of green beans), Kale, Onions, Sweet Peppers, Pumpkin, Rutabagas (another forgotten root worth rediscovering), Spinach, Squash, Sweet potatoes, Swiss chard, Tomatoes, Turnips, Watercress, and many, many more. Bon Appétit!

Alain's other vegetable recipes: *Alain's Healthy Green Soup, page 182. Carrots, Carrot Grens and Sweet Potato Soup, page 183. Spring Vegetable Minestrone, page 192. Gazpacho Soup, page 195. Cold Beet Soup with Yogurt, page 197. Cold Spinach and Avocado Soup, page 198. Oven-roasted Rosemary New potatoes, page 204. Roasted Haricots Verts with Hazelnuts, page 207. Ratatouille, page 208. Mixed Field Greens Salad with Grapefruit and Croutons, page 239. Niçoise Salad, page 240. Radicchio, Blood Orange, Arugula and Olive Salad, page 243. Asparagus, Garden Herbs and Parmesan Salad, page 244. Arugula, Cavaillon Melon and Serrano Ham Salad, page 245. Mixed Field Greens with Concord Pear, Walnuts and Roquefort, page 246. Grated Celeriac Salad with Yogurt Dressing, page 247. Carrot, Pineapple and Raisins Salad, page 249. Baby Spinach Salad with Fresh Raspberries and Almonds, page 250.*

Fruits. *Fruits*

Pommes. *Apples*

Please follow the same general shopping guidelines as in the vegetable chapter.

Apples originated in central Asia, specifically Kazakhstan. They were known 3,000 years ago in China, via the Silk Road, and thanks to Greek and Roman merchant ships, they eventually came to Europe. They then arrived in America with the European settlers near Boston. Some people claim that the fruit that Eve offered to Adam was not an apple - it was a quince. There! The record is set straight for America's favorite fruit.

I'm sure you know the old proverb "An apple a day keeps the doctor away". It turns out that popular wisdom has it right: apples should be a frequent addition to your diet. Maybe not every day, but at least 2 to 3 times a week. It has been found that an apple a day lowers the chance of heart attack by 32% in men at risk.

How do they help? For one thing, apples are loaded with antioxidants. Apples contain a wide assortment of phytochemicals such as *quercetin* (very helpful for heart health), *catechin, phloridzin* and *chlorogenic* acid, all powerful antioxidants. Apples also contain flavonoids, part of the polypherol family, are both antioxidants and anti-inflammatory. By the way, all of these beneficial phytonutrients are found primarily in the skin so make sure to wash your apple well and eat it with the skin on. Next to cranberries, apples contain the most antioxidants of the common fruits.

Do you remember that beneficial fiber I talked about earlier? Well, it turns out that apples are loaded with it. The skin provides insoluble fiber that, like bran, attaches to cholesterol in our digestive tract and help remove it from our body. They also contain pectin, a soluble fiber that can help us lower the bad cholesterol levels (LDL) in our liver. Apples contain an average of 5 g of fiber. Enjoy an apple every day if you can.

Alain's shopping advice

My favorite French variety is the Reine des Reinettes with its sweet acidity. It works very well in baked apple tarts. In America, the Granny Smith is my favorite baking apple and the one I like to eat raw is the Royal Gala. Normandy and Brittany are famous for their fermented apple cider (cidre bouché). For juice, instead of drinking commercial "apple juice" which is loaded with sugar and contains no live enzymes, I would prefer if you use a juice extractor to get the health benefits of freshly extracted apple juice. Bar that, try to find an organic apple juice that has not been pasteurized – probably coming from a local orchard.

Alain's cooking tips

Most of the time, I prefer to eat my apples "au naturel". That's the best way to get all the health benefit this tempting fruit has to offer. On special occasions, I prepare a "compote de pommes" (applesauce) or a "tarte aux pommes" (apple tart).

I always buy organic apples. Being such a popular fruit has made the price very reasonable. Since regular apples are on the list of fruits having the most pesticide residue, why go any other way? Pick a firm apple with bright colors. If there is a slight defect, as long as it's not marked or shriveled, it will be fine. Sometimes, organic apples don't look as perfect as regular apples, but I will take slight imperfection over pesticide-loaded perfection any day.

<u>**Alain's Recipes**</u>: *Baked Pork Chops with Apples and Cinnamon, page 222. Baked Apples with French Whipped Cream, page 255.*

Avocats. *Avocados*

I know, this fruit is not considered a staple of French food, but recently, French chefs have adopted this delicious and healthy fruit as one of their own. In France, our avocados come mostly from Israel. Also, the fact that I live in Texas has a large influence on my choice as well. How could I not mention guacamole? But, in addition to being delicious and a local food staple, avocados contain a type of fat that is beneficial to our cholesterol levels. Yes, avocados contain fats, but they are of the good-for-you variety called monounsaturated fats. They also contain a type of omega-9 fat called oleic acid that can be also found in Mediterranean ingredients such as olive oil, macadamia oil, walnut oil and other nuts. Monounsaturated fats are known to lower cholesterol.

In a study done by the Mexican Health Department, volunteers that ate avocados every day saw their total cholesterol levels drop by 17%. But wait, there's more! The interesting part is that their cholesterol ratio improved. Their levels of LDL (bad) cholesterol and triglycerides dropped while their levels of HDL (good) cholesterol went up. Remember, this is what we're trying to accomplish through this program. Lower our bad cholesterol and triglycerides levels and increase our levels of protective HDL cholesterol. Eating avocados regularly is one way to do that. Also, avocados provide a good amount of a plant substance called beta-sitosterol, known to significantly lower blood cholesterol. Let's not forget their fiber content, which can be between 11 and 17 g per avocado, depending on size.

Alain's shopping advice

The way I prefer to buy my avocados is unripe (hard to the touch) and allow them to ripen at home at ambient room temperature or, if you wish to accelerate the process, in a brown paper bag. If you're in a hurry, buy avocados that give slightly to gentle pressure of your thumb.

Alain's cooking tips

As a single man, I like to keep things simple at home. I slice it in half lengthwise. With a knife, I pry out the seed and throw it away. I then cut slices inside the fruit shell and again crosswise and drizzle it with my favorite salad dressing and scoop it out with a spoon. Other times, I will add the cut avocado to a mixed green salad, dress it with my favorite vinaigrette and toss it lightly.

Alain's Recipes: *Cold Spinach and Avocado Soup, page 198. Avocado Sauce, page 253.*

Myrtilles ou Bleuets. *Blueberries*

In France, we call them myrtilles and they are usually picked from wild bushes. That's the way I used to know them when I was raised on my grandparent's farm. We did not find them on the farm, but we would trade other foods for them at the local farmer's market. That's the best way you can have them, freshly picked in season. Bar that, cultivated blueberries are a very good source of antioxidants and fruit fiber. They rate as one of the highest of all fresh fruits in the ORAC (Oxygen Radical Absorbance Capacity) test. Antioxidants prevent free radical damage to your body especially in your arteries where oxidized cholesterol deposits as plaque and can lead to atherosclerosis. They also contain a compound called pterostilbene that shows an ability to regulate fatty acids in the bloodstream and help prevent plaque deposits in our arteries. They are also known as eye and memory food. So, sprinkle them over your breakfast oatmeal or salads and enjoy not only their health attributes, but also their wonderful flavor.

Alain's shopping advice

If possible, buy in season from local suppliers. Look for deep, dark blue, plump fruits. The bottom absorbent material should be free of stains. When home, take them out of the container and take out any unripe, moldy or wrinkled berries.

Alain's cooking tips

The simpler, the better. I like to sprinkle them on my morning cereal, mix them in my plain yogurt sweetened with a little local honey or added to my mixed greens salad to add an extra touch of antioxidants. They are delicious in any kind of fruit salad.

Alain's Recipes: *Blueberry Pecan Pancakes, page 168. A Votre Santé Healthy Home-made Breakfast Cereal, page 172. Fruit Salad with Fresh Ginger Dressing, page 259.*

Figues. *Figs*

In the South of France, you don't have to look very far to find figs hanging from trees. They are everywhere, even when I lived in an apartment, I did not have to go very far to find them in my neighbor's garden. (Just don't tell him I used to "borrow" his figs! Besides, they were hanging over the fence, so they were public property, right? They were still warm from the sun and very tasty, not to mention free.) Figs are also a wonderful snack when eaten dried. If you have blood sugar issues, you can use dried fig puree as a natural sweetener.

Figs are a very good source of fiber. Four to six fresh figs contain 5 g of soluble fiber. And they taste great to boot. What more would you want? That's the whole purpose of this book: live a healthy life while enjoying foods that taste great as they are keeping you healthy.

Alain's shopping advice

In the South of France, figs are easy to find, but it's a little more difficult in Texas. I wait until the beginning of the season (June to October) and look for my favorite, Black Mission figs. They are deep purple on the outside with a bright red flesh inside. I try to buy them ripe. I avoid those that are hard, mushy, or show signs of mold. I am gentle with them as their skin is very fragile and they bruise and rot quickly. If not quite ripe, I will let them ripen at home at room temperature, single layered on a plate covered with paper towel. When ripe, they should be tender to the touch and smell sweet. They can keep two to three days in your refrigerator but I would suggest you eat them at room temperature.

Alain's cooking tips

This is another case where simpler is better. I cut mine in quarters and savor them as is, full of flavor. At Moulin de Mougins, we would quarter them and drizzle them with crème fraîche. The contrast between the slight sourness of the unsweetened cream and the fig's sweetness was heaven. Nothing else was needed.

Pamplemousse. *Grapefruit*

Grapefruit is another fruit that is not indigenous to the South of France, but since it comes from a Mediterranean country (Israel), I include it here. Besides, it does provide health benefits for people with high triglycerides. In a study conducted in Israel, a group of patients with high triglyceride levels were split into three groups: one group was given the standard "heart healthy" diet, the second was given the same heart healthy diet plus white grapefruits, and the third was also given the heart healthy diet but ate Jaffa red grapefruits instead. The group who ate the diet complemented with red grapefruits lowered their LDL (bad) cholesterol levels by 20 percent. A very impressive result considering these same patients had previously been on cholesterol-lowering drugs and showed no noticeable positive results. The main reason for these different results is that red grapefruits have a higher content of antioxidants than white grapefruits. Jaffa grapefruits are difficult to find here in America, but here in Texas we have access to the wonderful Ruby Red grapefruits from the Rio Grande Valley.

Alain's shopping advice

I prefer my grapefruit to be smallish with a bright smooth skin. I never quite understood the appeal of giant grapefruits. Unfailingly, they turn out to have a thick skin and mealy meat. Grapefruits should be very heavy for their size with a thin skin that springs back to the touch. It should not be soft. If they have the above qualities with a few skin defects, pick them anyway; they will be good.

Grapefruit does not continue to ripen after being harvested. You can keep them at room temperature for a few days until ready to eat them. Otherwise, store them in your vegetable crisper and they will last longer, but be sure to allow them to come back to room temperature before you savor them.

Alain's cooking tips

I like to eat them just as they are with a teaspoon. Sometimes, if I feel fancy, I will sprinkle a little bit of raw sugar on top and broil them to add a caramel flavor to their sweetness. They are a wonderful addition to any fruit salad. If possible, try to cut the meat between the partitions so you don't have to deal with the bitter skin.

Alain's Recipes: *Mixed Field Greens Salad with Grapefruit and Croutons, page 239. Red Grapefruit and Orange Salad, page 258.*

Raisins. *Grapes*

You probably all know that France is one of the most prolific wine producers in the world. But that's not what I'm talking about here; grapes alone are not only very good to eat, but good for your cholesterol.

Grapes contain a compound called resveratrol which the plant creates to protect itself from dangerous microorganisms, but it is also beneficial to we humans as well. It is a powerful antioxidant. High intake of resveratrol in red wine and grape skin is known to reduce cardiovascular diseases. The skins of dark grapes are the best source of resveratrol.

Another beneficial compound is OPC (oligomeric proanthocyanidins). Proanthocyanidins are part of the flavonoids family and are powerful antioxidants, many times more effective than vitamins C and E. Several studies have shown that OPCs can help reduce the negative effect of high cholesterol in our body. A recent study in Spain showed that people drinking about half a cup of fresh red grape juice (not the bottled stuff) showed a significantly lower LDL (bad) cholesterol levels and increased HDL (good) cholesterol levels. It also showed a decrease in inflammatory markers, which are an indication for free radical damages.

To make it easier, I would suggest you eat 4 ounces of red organic grapes per sitting, especially if you're concerned about the blood sugar levels. If you cannot find organic grapes, make sure to wash them thoroughly.

Alain's shopping advice

There are 2 main varieties of table grapes: European and Native. European grapes were brought to America by French, Italian, German, and even English immigrants. There is Thompson (amber-green and seedless), Emperor (purple and seeded), and Champagne/Black Corinth (purple and tiny, more difficult to find, as they are used mostly dried as Zante currants).

European grapes have a skin that adheres closely to the flesh. Thompson grapes are the best known of the three and my favorite. I also love to get champagne grapes when in season.

The Native American grapes are the Concord (blue-black, seeded and large), Delaware (pink-red, seeded), and Niagara (amber colored and seeded). Concord grapes are mostly used for juice and jellies. Native American grapes have skins that can be peeled easily.

When I was a kid, I used to love seeded grapes I could spit out and have contests with my friends. These days, I'm just as happy with the seedless variety.

Alain's cooking tips

To eat them as is, just rinse them under cold water and pat dry. Instead of ice cream, a sweet and natural treat for kids is frozen grapes. Pick a seedless variety. After washing them, separate them on a tray covered with paper towel and freeze. When frozen, store them in a resealable plastic bag and enjoy them while watching your favorite movie at home.

Alain's Recipes: *Chicken Salad with Grapes and Toasted Walnuts, page 228.*

Citrons et Citrons Verts. *Lemons and Limes*

Now, there is a crop that the Cote d'Azur can be proud of. Lemons and oranges are a prolific crop in the South of France. So much so that there is a famous Lemon Carnival every year on Mardi Gras in the city of Menton, about 10 miles East of my hometown of Nice. Huge floats are created but instead of "papier mâché" characters like in New Orleans and Nice, they are covered with lemons, limes and oranges grown in the region. A couple of times as a teenager, I would jump on my moped and travel to Menton to be amazed at the colorful display of citrus fruits.

Of course, you already know that citrus fruits are loaded with vitamin C, a known antioxidant. But what you may not know is that their skin contains two powerful phytochemicals known as limonoids: limonene and limonin. While limonene is respected as an anti-cancer phytochemical, it seems that limonin helps lower cholesterol. So there you have it, antioxidant protection and cholesterol-lowering properties. Did you know that a cube of sugar soaked with lemon juice is an infallible remedy for hiccup? The effect is immediate and is very safe.

Alain's shopping advice

There are lemons (*Citrus Limon*) and there are limes. Although they are both from the same *citrus* family, they are cousins, not brothers. Limes are not green lemons, they are *Citrus aurantifolia*. What I'm looking for when picking lemons and limes is a tight, shiny and thin skin. They should feel heavy and spring back when pressed gently. I love to use key limes for a real key lime pie but could never get used to the sweet flavor of the Meyer lemon. For me, a lemon or a lime should taste sour.

Alain's cooking tips

To take advantage of their healthy properties, use organic lemons to make fresh lemonade. Don't forget to use the peel as well. If you feel adventurous and own one of those powerful blenders like Vita-Mix, I would suggest you use the whole fruit. Another way to use the peel is by adding a sliver of it to your espresso like the Italians do, or add a lemon slice in your tea as the English do. I personally always drink my water with a quarter of lime squeezed into it. It's a good way to help reduce the chance of kidney stones.

Of course, there are plenty of other uses for lemons and limes. I like to squeeze half a lime on my fish. I love fresh lemon and lime curd. Here are a few recipes:

Alain's Recipes: *Lemon Cream Sauce, page 254. Tarts with English Lemon Curd and French Meringue, page 262.*

Olives. *Olives*

As you might imagine, olives were part of my upbringing. You might be surprised to hear that when I was a kid, I refused to eat the black olives that came with my pizza. My mother used to make fun of me: "How can you live in Nice and not like olives?" Well, that was then and this is now. I now love olives for their taste and their health benefits. Mind you, I'm a little picky; if possible, I try to get the Olives Niçoises (olives from Nice). Not only because they come from my hometown, but because they are still cured the old-fashioned way, in a "saumure" (brine) made of spring water and sea salt. They are good for your digestive health, because they are one of the naturally fermented foods full of active cultures I mentioned earlier. That should be the only way of preparing olives, but as you can guess, the vast majority of commercial olives are not cured this way. I am not a big fan of other types of olives, processed or not. I don't care for green olives; I'm sure they're good (if handled properly), they're just not for me. Olives provide us with the same health benefits as olive oil, plus fiber.

Alain's shopping advice

If your grocery store has an olive bar, as Whole Foods Market and Central Market do, by all means buy your olives there. You could be lucky and find "olives de Nice"! Otherwise, you should be able to find them at a Greek or Italian food market or store. Make sure to ask for naturally fermented olives.

Alain's cooking tips

Olives need little preparation. I like to use them on salads, easy homemade pizza, or just as is with a little goat cheese and toasted baguette slices. Yum!

<u>Alain's Recipes</u>: *Tapenade, page 177.*

Oranges. *Oranges*

Another proud fruit from the South of France. Like lemons and limes, oranges contain a large amount of the phytochemical called *limonoids*. Some of the benefits being investigated at this time are limonoids' antiviral, antifungal, antibacterial as well as anti-neoplastic and anti-malarial properties. That's a lot of beneficial qualities from a fruit we tend to take for granted! As a matter of fact, at my house, I only use an orange peel-based all-purpose cleaner after throwing away all my other potentially toxic cleaners. It smells wonderful and reminds me of the fragrance floating in the Cote d'Azur air. I know, I'm being a little too sentimental, but that's how I fight my homesickness.

Another flavonoid contained in the orange's skin is *hesperidin*. It is a proven anti-inflammatory as well as being vasoprotective (protects your blood vessels). To top it off, it has anti-allergic and anti-carcinogenic properties. Combined with their natural vitamin C content, *hesperidin* helps lower our LDL (bad) cholesterol and increase our HDL (good) cholesterol.

By the way, do not think that by drinking your commercially-squeezed orange juice every morning, you're doing yourself a favor. Not only are processed juices loaded with sugar, they are also pasteurized, which negates many of orange juice's beneficial qualities. Please, if you want orange juice in the morning, squeeze it yourself. It will do you more good, and will not affect your blood sugar levels the way the commercial versions will.

Alain's shopping advice

Like lemons and limes, oranges are part of the citrus family. The sweet orange we eat usually is called *Citrus sinensis* and is different from the bitter orange (*Citrus aurantium)* used for English-style orange marmalade. Like lemons, limes and grapefruits, look for a firm fruit with thin skin.

Alain's cooking tips

I prefer them just the way they come, peeled and quartered. I also love them in a fruit salad with a touch of Grand Marnier to accentuate the orange flavor. I add the zest and juice to my cranberry sauce, and I also make a mean orange Grand Marnier crepe.

Alain's Recipes: *Orange Grand Marnier French Crêpes, page 260.*

Pruneaux. *Prunes*

In my opinion, prunes have been made fun of for too long. First of all, because they're loaded with fiber, they are helpful to our intestinal transit. They are also loaded with health-supporting phytonutrients called phenolics. The phenolics in prunes are *neochlorogenic acid* and *chlorogenic acid,* two powerful antioxidants very effective against those nasty free radicals that damage our cells and make us age faster. In the ORAC test I mentioned before, they rank twice as high as blueberries and raisins.

It is said that the special plums used to make prunes were brought back from the crusades after the siege of Damas in Syria. The best-known French variety of plums is called plums d'Ente. Since they were mostly grown near the town of Agen, they came to be known as Prunes d'Agen. They were imported to America by a Frenchman named Louis Pellier in 1856. American production is centered in California, the world's largest producer of prunes. I bet you did not know you owed your regularity to a Frenchman.

Alain's shopping advice

If possible, buy them bulk and organic, but since they are typically not heavily sprayed with pesticides, regular prunes will do just fine.

Alain's cooking tips

My experience with prunes began when I was a pastry chef in a health resort and offered poached prunes in red wine and "cannelle" (cinnamon) on "ma carte des desserts" (the dessert menu). I don't care about what some snickering people will say; they are a wonderful dessert. When eaten as a snack with a raw almond, it's a perfect natural pick-me-up loaded with healthy fibers, sugars and monounsaturated fats, all good for your cholesterol levels.

Alain's Recipes: *Roasted Turkey with Prunes and Apples, page 230. Red Wine and Cinnamon Prunes Compote, page 261.*

Kaki. *Persimmons*

Although this fruit is probably unknown to you, it is recently been recognized as a very healthful fruit. It originated in East China, is the national fruit of Japan and is cultivated all around the Mediterranean basin, including the South of France. When I was a kid roaming the streets, I would grab one and bite into it. Big mistake! If it is not perfectly ripe to the point of rotting, its tannin content makes it a very bitter fruit indeed.

Persimmons are loaded with vitamin A and carotenoids, and also contain a good amount of soluble fiber. In an Israeli lab test, rats fed with persimmons showed a much lower LDL (bad) cholesterol and triglyceride levels as well as lower lipid peroxides (a measure of cholesterol oxidation in the blood). They are also a good source of iron, potassium, magnesium and manganese.

So, if you feel adventurous, I encourage you to try this fruit, as long as you make sure it is very ripe. You can help the maturing of this fruit by placing it in a paper bag as you would bananas.

Alain's shopping advice

There are two types of persimmons: astringent (Hachiya or Japanese persimmon) and non-astringent (Fuyu). More difficult to find is the Sharon fruit (Israel persimmon) that, like the Fuyu, is non-astringent. Both of these can be eaten any time you wish. They tend to be crunchy like apples. From my personal experience, I still find the Hachiya tastier than the other varieties.

Alain's cooking tips

The best way to eat them is to cut them in half and scoop the pulp out with a spoon.

Autres Fruits. *Other Fruits*

Of course, I could not possibly list every fruit. I have focused on the ones that are proven to have a beneficial effect on cholesterol levels. But, to repeat myself, all fruits are loaded with soluble fiber and antioxidants, some more than others. Eat at least two fresh fruits a day, in season, and enjoy your lower cholesterol.

Other Fruits Recipes: *Raspberry Muffins, page 169. Cranberry Scones with Walnut Pieces, page 170. Fruit Salad with Fresh Ginger Dressing, page 259. Fredericksburg Peach Sorbet, page 266. Light as a Cloud Raspberry Soufflé, page 256.*

Fruits Secs et Graines Assorties. *Assorted Nuts and Seeds*

As a group, nuts and seeds should be regular additions to our diet. They are a good source of fiber, and most of the fat they contain is monounsaturated fat, known to be beneficial to our health. In the US, the Nurse's Health Study of about 35,000 women has shown a 30 to 50 percent lower risk of heart disease for the ladies that eat nuts several times a week. One of the reasons may be due to an amino acid called *arginine*. *Arginine* makes our arterial walls more pliable by increasing the amount of nitric acid, a very important molecule believed to help relax constricted blood vessels and increase blood flow to our organs. It is credited with a lower susceptibility to atherosclerosis.

In the supplement world, arginine is considered to be the natural equivalent to Viagra. Nuts are very easy to incorporate into your daily diet, from adding them to your morning breakfast to sprinkling them on salads or eating them as a healthy snack. Again, don't overdo it. Moderation is the word.

Eat nuts raw to avoid damaging their fragile oils; do not roast nuts and seeds at high temperature as the high heat will oxidize the healthy oils they contain into trans-fatty acids. If you wish, you can still roast your nuts at 220°F for 20 to 30 minutes. That's the way I roast my tamari-coated almonds, a wonderful snack. So go nuts and munch on them – in moderation. They will return the favor with lower cholesterol levels.

Amandes et Beurre d'Amandes *Almonds and Almond Butter*

Almonds are my favorite snack. They're loaded with fiber and healthy monounsaturated oils. Besides that, the FDA (yes, even them) approved of eating almonds in the following cautious statement: "Scientific evidence suggests, but does not prove, that eating 1.5 ounces per day of most nuts, such as almonds, as a part of a diet low in saturated fat and cholesterol, may reduce the risk of heart disease." That's good enough for me. But wait, there is more!

I found an analysis on a Meta research that showed that people with high cholesterol eating almonds regularly showed a 5.3 to 7.2 decrease in total cholesterol levels and, to make it even more interesting, lowered their LDL (bad) cholesterol from 6.8 to 10 percent.

Alain's shopping advice

Buy them organic and raw. Avoid buying dry roasted almonds as the roasting process damages their fragile oils. The worst is oil-fried, like the kind that comes in a can with the top hat character on it. Not only is the oil used in the process damaged by countless overheating, but the high heat damages the almonds as well. Double whammy! Just as bad as deep-frying a hamburger.

Alain's cooking tips

I usually either toss whole almonds with an organic tamari sauce and roast them at a low temperature, or I eat them with unsulfured dried apricots as a healthy snack. That way, I get my protein and fiber as well as some fruit sugar from the apricot. I also love to spread almond butter on a Swedish grain cracker and top it off with my favorite raspberry preserves.

Alain's Recipes: *Trout Filets Amandine, page 238. Cocoa and Almond Meringues, page 263.*

Noix de Cajou. *Cashew Nut*

Cashew nuts basically have the same benefits as almonds and other nuts; they provide you with loads of fiber and healthy monounsaturated fats.

Alain's shopping advice

Again, buy them raw and toast them lightly if you feel like it. It's much healthier for you that way. Also, try to buy at a store with high volume so the nuts don't have time to turn rancid and oxidize.

Alain's cooking tips

Toast them lightly at 220°F for about 20 minutes. If you want you can sprinkle them with crushed sea salt. Raw cashews make wonderful cashew butter. Try it as an alternative to peanut butter.

Noisettes. *Hazelnuts, Filberts*

I honestly don't understand why hazelnuts are so under-appreciated in this country. They have a wonderfully subtle flavor that goes particularly well with chocolate, as in Nutella. In Europe, they are mostly grown in Northern Italy and that's where the famous Gianduja chocolate comes from, a blend of hazelnut butter and milk chocolate. If you have never had it, you don't know what you're missing. In this country, the closest thing you can find would be in the chocolate Rocher by Ferrero.

Hazelnuts provide the same benefits as other nuts, plus another interesting ingredient: beta-sitosterol, which is found in pecans as well. Beta-sisterol is a plant sterol that is credited with two important properties: it lowers cholesterol and it reduces the symptoms of prostatic hyperplasia some men experience as they age. Another little known advantage is that they contain a decent amount of omega-3 fatty acids. Now, if that does not make you rush to the store and try poor unloved hazelnuts, I don't know what will.

Alain's shopping advices

Buy them organic, in bulk, at a high-volume store.

Alain's cooking tips

I love to add lightly toasted and chopped hazelnuts to my mixed green salad. And, in my opinion, hazelnut butter is a better and healthier alternative to peanut butter, which, by the way, is almost unknown in Europe.

Cacahuètes et Beurre de Cacahuètes. *Peanuts and Peanut Butter*

I know what I said above and I stand by my position, but that does not mean that you have to throw away your jar of peanut butter – unless it contains trans fatty acids and hydrogenated fats. Peanuts (which, by the way, is not really a nut but a legume) are still a healthy addition to your cholesterol-lowering diet. They contain a good amount of fiber and has a special polyphenol called *p-coumaric acid*. P-coumaric acid is a powerful antioxidant. Not only that, but it was found that roasting the peanuts would increase their content of p-coumaric acid by up to 22 percent.

Wait, there's more good news: in another study conducted at Penn State University, it was found that people making a point of eating peanuts or peanut butter daily experienced a 13 percent decrease in their triglycerides levels. It also contains about 50 percent high-oleic acid monounsaturated fat, which, just like olive oil, has been found to be beneficial in the Lyon's Mediterranean Diet Study.

Alain's cooking tips

To be honest with you, probably because I'm French, I'm not a peanut butter fan for reasons of taste. It's a cultural thing I guess, especially since there are so many other wonderful nut alternatives out there. Nope, don't even try to convince me, I won't touch the stuff.

But that should not stop you. But whatever you do, do NOT use the type loaded with sugar and hydrogenated fats. Buy peanut butter at your local health store. Better yet, some stores provide a grinder where you can grind your own fresh peanut butter.

Noix de Pecan. *Pecan Nuts*

Living in Texas it's hard to avoid pecans. They're everywhere in every shape and form you can imagine. It is not a typical crop in France (unlike walnuts), but lately, creative chefs there have adopted it too.

Like all nuts, they contain a good amount of fiber (3 g per serving of about 20 pecan halves) and monounsaturated oil. And like hazelnuts, they contain beta-sitosterol, a plant sterol known to lower cholesterol.

Alain's shopping advice

Like walnuts, if you don't mind the extra work, shell them yourself and enjoy them at the peak of freshness and nutrition.

Alain's cooking tips

I like to eat them as a snack with dried fruits. You can enjoy them dry-roasted but I prefer them raw. You can also make pecan butter (again, raw is best), or toss them with your favorite salad or breakfast cereals. They are also a good addition to a healthy smoothie.

Pistaches. *Pistachio Nuts*

Here is another memory floating to the surface: for a while, in my hometown of Nice on the Cote d'Azur, I worked for an Italian ice cream maker. Amongst all the different flavors of gelato offered, one of my favorites was pistachio. Typically, I would sneak a finger into a batch to savor it the guilty way. When I did it the right way, I got a scoop and covered it with chocolate sauce. Double yum! Pistachio ice cream is harder to find in the US, but if you live in a big city, there's bound to be a gelato store somewhere in town. So go and enjoy my treat the way I did... just know it's not the healthy way to eat pistachios.

In the good-for-you department, pistachios have been found to improve total and HDL (good) cholesterol levels and decrease oxidative stress. They also helped improve the total cholesterol to HDL ratio by 21 percent. This ration is considered to be an important ratio to watch for your cardiovascular health.

They also contain a good amount of plant phytosterols (270 mg per 100 g serving) known for their positive effect on cholesterol metabolism. Pistachios are much better for you when eaten out of the shell.

Alain's shopping advice

Do not buy the red-colored type. Some creative guy came up with this idea one day and apparently people got fooled into believing it's a better quality of pistachios. It's not, it's only artificial coloring so pass on it. Also, be cautious about salt content. If you can, buy them dry-roasted with no or very little added salt.

Noix. Walnuts

Walnuts are so important in French diet that they gave it a name that means nuts in French as if they were the only nuts around. Believe me, there are plenty of nuts around, but that's another issue.

To get back to walnuts, have you ever noticed how, when shelled and separated in two halves, they look like a miniature brain? Well, there is a centuries-old theory called the Doctrine of Signatures that posit that some foods look like the organ they're supposed to help. So, there you have it, walnuts are good for your brain... and your heart as well. How so? They are the nuts containing the largest amount of cholesterol-friendly omega-3 fatty acids. Amongst many other benefits, omega-3 fatty acids are known to lower triglycerides and reduce plaque formation.

Do you remember me mentioning the AOC certification system I talked about in the lentils paragraph? Well, theses walnuts are so full of themselves, they are labeled AOC in not one, but two regions in France: Grenoble and Perigord. How about that? That's how important we think they are. Apparently our French Cro-Magnon ancestors like them so much, walnuts were found in historical digs. In the middle ages, their oil was used as lighting oil and was the only cheap source of oil for the poor peasants living in the region.

Alain's shopping advices

Like pecans, they are much healthier for you when shelled fresh. You can find them like that in the autumn. Bar that, organic or not should not matter much in this case. Use halves or pieces, your choice.

Alain's cooking tips

In France walnuts have many uses. First of all, they make a very delicate and flavorful dressing salad oil. Please never cook with this oil as it is a polyunsatured fat, which is very healthy but degrades very fast when heated. They are also used in cooking, baking and also as a walnut butter, just like peanut butter only better (can you tell I'm not quite impartial here?). It's also a very good source of easy protein when blended in your favorite smoothie. I also like them as an afternoon snack with a dried fruit like apricot or a spoonful of raisins. I use them in my grape raisin chicken salad.

Alain's Recipes: *Tender Walnut Muffins, page 171. Chicken Salad with Grapes and Toasted Walnuts, page 228.*

Graines Assorties. *Assorted Seeds*

Graines de Citrouille. *Pumpkin Seeds*

When I was a kid and my Grand-mere was making a "soupe de citrouille" (pumpkin soup), I had no clue how beneficial the seeds were for our health. Now I know. Pumpkin seeds contain beta-sitosterol, less than pecans and hazelnuts but enough to help lower our cholesterol and ease prostatic hyperplasia. They also have a respectable amount of phytosterols of 265 mg per 100 g serving; less than pistachios, but still helpful.

Alain's cooking tips

I personally mix them in both my morning breakfast cereal and my tamari-roasted nut mix. You can eat them raw or dry-roasted. Both versions contain a good amount of magnesium, potassium and phosphorus.

<u>Alain's Recipes</u>: *Alain's famous oatmeal breakfast p 172.*

Graines et Beurre de Sésame (Tahini). *Sesame Seeds, Sesame Butter, also called Tahini*

Sesame seeds are not used very often in France unless they are part of a recipe in a Middle Eastern restaurant. Since we have a lot of them in the South of France, I do not feel out of line including them here. Amongst many other benefits, sesame seeds are a good source of cholesterol-reducing phytosterols. As I mentioned above, beta-sitosterol is known to lower cholesterol. As a matter of fact, they contain 400 mg per 100 g of beta-sitosterol. The same as wheat-germ! They are in good company indeed.

Sesame seeds also contain a generous amount of *lignans*. Lignans are one of the major classes of phytoestrogens, a form of plant estrogen found in flax seeds and sesame seeds. Lignans are also recognized as antioxidants. *Sesamin*, one of the forms of lignans used in a study published in the *Journal of Lipid Research* have been shown to lower blood serum cholesterol as well as liver cholesterol levels. There is a lot of promise in these little seeds.

In another study conducted with healthy postmenopausal women, sesame seed powder was ingested for five weeks and showed an improvement in LDL (bad) cholesterol levels, total to HDL cholesterol ratio and antioxidant levels.

Alain's shopping advice

If you can find them organic, more power to you. Buy from a high volume store and they will be less likely to have oxidized.

Graines de Tournesol. *Sunflower Seeds*

Sunflower seeds contain a good amount of fiber (4 g per serving) and our old friend, beta-sitosterol, a phytosterol known for its ability to lower cholesterol levels and help with prostate health. Sunflower seeds and pistachio nuts contain the highest amount of these friendly phytosterols. These seeds are loaded with zinc, which is good for your immune system and protects against prostate cancer. They are also filled with the powerful antioxidants selenium and vitamin E.

Alain's shopping advice

Buy them raw and organic, if possible.

Produits Laitiers and Eggs. *Dairy Products and Eggs*

I know, some people will say« il est fou ce gars » (this guy's crazy), but there are good reasons to include some dairy products in this book. Unlike a lot of nutritionists and probably because I'm French, a reasonable amount (remember, moderation) of properly handled dairy products will not kill you. It might actually make you feel good after tasting some of these wonderful French cheeses now available in this country.

The difference is how are these products handled and processed. I hate to talk about the good old days, but in this case, they had it right. Increasingly in this country, local farms are going back to the old ways in order to offer quality dairy products that are properly made. I will not go into a complicated debate here, and I also know that I will not be able to convince the vast majority of you, but if you'd rather not read this, just skip the dairy section and everyone will be happy.

To make a long story short, dairy products should be coming from grass-fed cows, which produce omega-3-rich milk, cream and cheese. Once collected, dairy products should be minimally processed with no or low pasteurization and NO homogenization.

Dairy products should not come from feedlots where the poor cows are crowded and riddled with disease, injected with growth hormones and antibiotics, and are fed corn instead of grass (which creates products loaded with omega-6 fatty acids, known to be inflammatory). Oh, and the way they are "processed" (killed) is highly cruel and stressful to the cows which generates stress hormones in the meat. Are you disgusted yet? I know I am. This industrial way of producing dairy is destroying all the original qualities of what used to be wholesome products.

Dairy products do contain saturated fats. But you should know that most of us get only 25 percent of our cholesterol from food. Our body produces the rest. Besides, when you eat healthy saturated fats, it raises both your good and bad cholesterol. Some scientists even claim that it raises the good cholesterol more than the bad. We need to be reasonable about this whole low-fat hysteria. Eating a reasonable amount of saturated fat products like dairy, avocado and eggs is not going to kill you and most likely is healthy for you (again in moderation). I personally eat cheese about once a week, avocados a couple of times a week and an egg every day.

To be clear with you, since I am lactose intolerant, I do not drink cows milk. I drink soy, almond, hazelnut, or hemp milk and they work for me. You can also drink rice milk if you choose. On the other hand, I could not live without my beautiful French cheese. But I only occasionally eat a small piece, savored with a nice slice of "pain de campagne" (country-style whole wheat bread). That's a special treat for me and that is how it should be enjoyed, with no guilt. Pleasure in moderation is much better than guilty pleasure. I also eat plain, naturally fermented yogurt (White Mountain Brand, made in Austin) since the friendly bacteria in the yogurt have already digested the lactose. And yogurt is helpful to your digestive system, as are most naturally fermented products.

Ultimately, the choice is yours and I respect that. Do what feels right for you but, if you're curious about it, do your own research at www.westonaprice,org. They offer a lot of good articles explaining why we shouldn't consume modern dairy products. You may choose to ignore their advice and believe the milk-mustachioed celebrities, but at least you'll be informed.

Lait Frais. *Fresh Milk*

Alain's shopping advice

It is very difficult to find fresh raw milk, as it is illegal to sell or even purchase raw milk in many states. It is possible, but not easy. Otherwise, buy whole organic milk from **Organic Valley**.

Alain's cooking tips

As raw milk has not been pasteurized, it will not keep as long as conventional pasteurized/homogenized milk.

Fromage. *Cheese*

Growing up, the local unpasteurized cheeses were wonderful to eat, even though we could only afford them once in a rare while. That made the cheese even more precious. I would savor each tiny bite. It was nothing like what passes for cheese in most American grocery stores. Luckily for us, the past 20 years have seen a tremendous increase of cheeses from all parts of the world in America. When I came to this country thirty years ago, you could find a few rare choices at Dean and Delucca, or Zabars in New York City. Things have changed for the better since then. When I can find it, I prefer to eat unpasteurized cheese, mostly from local farms. You can find them at your local farmer's market or check online for a reputable source in your area.

Alain's shopping advices

Wow! This is a very complicated subject. As you may know, in France only, we have more cheese types than there are days in a year. So I'm going to keep it really simple. Buy local! If you're lucky enough to have raw or lightly pasteurized cheese produced in your region, enjoy.

Alain's cooking tips

Nope, you can't really cook with it. Oops! I almost forgot "Brie en Croute" (Brie in crust) or "Brie en Brioche" (Brie in brioche – a type of sweet French bread). Double oops! What about "fondue" and "raclette"? When I came to this country in the late 70s, there was a huge fad for everything fondue. Cheese fondue (bread and melted cheese), "fondue Bourguignonne" (beef cooked in oil then dipped in an assortment of sauces), even chocolate fondue (pieces of fruit dipped in chocolate). You could find fondue restaurants everywhere and a fondue set in every household worth its salt. What about now? Poof! All gone. Too bad, it was fun while it lasted.

I like to sprinkle Roquefort (a type of blue cheese) and walnut pieces over a green salad. It's a classic in France. Otherwise, I love pretty much any cheese (not just French) with a fresh piece of French baguette (in Austin, try Sweetish Hill, Phoenicia Bakery or Whole Foods Market downtown) and a good glass of red wine. A Votre Santé!

Alain's Recipes: *Melted Goat Cheese on Walnut Bread, page 179.*

Yaourt et Kéfir. *Yogurt and Kefir*

Do you remember reading stories about an ancient tribe living in the Bulgarian mountains that lived long and healthy lives? Why did they live so long? Of course, the first reason was they did not have access to "modern" industrialized food products. But the reason given was that their main food was yogurt (or yoghurt), a fermented milk product that tastes very sour. Nowadays, you can find yogurt in myriad different flavors and textures.

Yogurt's main benefit is the healthy bacteria it contains. Not only do they digest the lactose in milk to make it more digestible, but also the friendly bacteria (probiotics, which literally mean "for life") are indispensable to a healthy body. You see, I believe, as do many other nutritionists that our health starts in our guts. Probiotics help us digest our food, strengthen our immune system and also protect us from an overgrowth of *Candida Albicans* (a form of yeast) which, if not kept in check, will invade our body and create all sort of annoying afflictions like thrush and yeast infections. The most common friendly bacteria are *lactobacillus* and *bifidobacteria*. If you can find real Bulgarian-style yogurts, they contain a different strain of probiotics called *bulgaricus*. (Also called *b.bifidum* or *bifidobacteria*). That's what makes them taste sour. Bulgaricus are believed to have antiviral, antibacterial and antifungal properties.

The American Journal of Clinical Nutrition writes: "By maintaining a healthy gut flora, you'll prevent all kinds of diseases, especially chronic degenerative ones."

So instead of killing our friendly bacteria by abusing antibiotics, let's help them by sending reinforcements in the form of gut-friendly fermented foods like yogurt, kefir, and real sauerkraut (naturally fermented chopped cabbage leaves). Also, if you can find them, see if the yogurts you buy have the Live and Active Cultures (LAC) label. It's a sign that the manufacturer is providing living probiotics in its products.

Alain's shopping advice

Don't believe all the newfound hype about digestive yogurt claims. Although these claims are partially true, what they don't mention is that, most of the time, these yogurts are loaded with additional sweeteners, flavors and even artificial coloring. My best advice is to keep it simple. Buy it plain, Bulgarian-style if you can find it. A few brands come to mind. In Austin, buy **White Mountain**. They're local and the freshest you can find. Other good national brands are **Brown Cow** and **Stonyfield**. I don't recommend any other commercial brands.

Alain's cooking tips

The only form of yogurt I choose to eat is the whole milk plain yogurt. If I choose to add sweetness to my yogurt (which I don't do often), I will add locally harvested creamy honey or sugar-free fruit preserves. Sometimes, I even add nuts or seeds to add that extra crunch. You can also mix it with your cereal in the morning.

<u>Alain's Recipes:</u> *Grated Celeriac Salad with Yogurt Dressing, page 247.*

Oeufs. *Eggs*

Eggs are nature's perfect food. You may ask "Aren't eggs bad for your cholesterol?" For years the public has been told to avoid eggs, especially the high-cholesterol yolks. The egg scare started in the 1950s and 1960s, during a campaign condemning cholesterol. Most patients and doctors still hold fast to the idea that eggs are bad for you because of their high cholesterol content; even though hundreds of studies have shown that the amount of cholesterol we eat has very little influence on our cholesterol blood levels. More to the point, specific studies have shown that consuming moderate amounts of eggs does not even affect our blood cholesterol levels.

Egg yolks do contain cholesterol, but what has been conveniently overlooked is the fact that they are also one of the richest sources of *choline*, a component of *lecithin*, which many people have eliminated or reduced in their diet. Choline acts like a fat and cholesterol dissolver. It keeps the cholesterol in the egg moving through your bloodstream and doesn't allow it to accumulate on arterial walls. Lecithin breaks fats into small droplets and improves digestion. It also keeps cholesterol soluble, which keeps it moving in the bloodstream and helps prevent blockages or clots. Eggs are also rich in minerals, vitamins, and essential amino acids. (If you don't want to eat eggs daily, one easy way to get these benefits is to make a healthy smoothie with a tablespoon of soy lecithin every day).

Another important fact to know is that farm-raised, free-range or organic eggs from chickens feeding freely in the fields contain a higher amount of omega-3 fatty acids, which are good for your HDL cholesterol level.

In recent research at the Kansas State University, scientists found a new substance in eggs called (take a breath) *phosphatidylcholine* that was found to block any LDL (bad) cholesterol from entering our bloodstream.

When I went to the market to buy eggs as a boy, the farmers used to have a small candle (later a flashlight bulb) set in a metal box with an opening just large enough to sit each egg in it. That way you could tell how fresh they were by the size of the air pocket in them. The larger the air pocket, the older the eggs were. I would not be surprised to see those same boxes still used at the markets in small French villages.

Alain's shopping advice

If you can, buy farm-fresh, free-range and cage-free eggs from a producer you know. This is by far your best choice. In Austin, we can get this type of eggs from **Boggy Creek Farm**, **Louis Young's Farm**, **Soncrest Egg Co.**, and **Coyote Creek Farm**. Be aware that, in some cases, free-range does not mean a whole lot. The USDA allows any farm that has a little door available for the chickens to use to be free-range. So, cage-free is a better designation if you want to make sure those chickens actually scratch the earth, feed on earth worms and gravel (what did you think the shell was made of?) like at my grandmother's farm. Your next choice should be organic omega-3 eggs, then organic eggs like **Organic Valley**.

Alain's cooking tips

The best way to cook eggs so they are easy to digest are poached or soft boiled, like the British like to eat them. Why? The egg white needs to be fully cooked as it could cause biotin deficiency over time. On the other hand it should not be overcooked (as in fried) which creates carcinogens. The eggs yolk is a lot easier to digest when barely cooked (sunny side up) or still raw but warm. Hard-boiled eggs are much more difficult for your body to assimilate. By the way, scrambling your morning eggs exposes them to oxidation, so I try to avoid cooking them that way.

Here are three methods of cooking your eggs gently:

1. Poached in simmering water with a teaspoon of vinegar and a pinch of sea salt added. Both help the white to coagulate. Let the egg poach on one side for a minute, turn it around gently and finish cooking. Drain it on a paper towel. I like to add tomato sauce to mine.

2. What I call butter-poached. I learned this technique a long time ago from an English cookbook (they know a thing or two about eggs, these lads). I melt a pat of butter gently in an egg-poacher. When it is liquid, add your egg. Let it poach gently at low temperature. The way I like mine is with crushed sea salt on the white and cayenne pepper on the yolk. Sometimes, I use a touch of turmeric for its health benefits.

3. Soft-boiled eggs, another English technique we have adopted heartily in France, especially in the South. In the wild days before World War II, rich English society loved to spend their winters on the Cote d'Azur. They left us a few new cooking ideas. Bring your cooking water to a gentle boil, add your eggs carefully and cook for 3 minutes from the time you add the egg to the water. Take the eggs out gently and run under water for about 30 seconds to avoid overcooking. I like to eat mine with a little sea salt and black pepper and dip in long pieces of French baguettes cut finger-size.

Alain's Recipes: *Alain's Way of making a Potato Omelet, page 175. Fines Herbs Omelet with Goat Cheese, page 176. My « Mamie's » French Toasts, page 174.*

Viande. *Meat*

Viande de Boeuf, Bison, Cochon, Poulet, Agneau, et Chevreuil. *Beef, Bison, Pork, Chicken, Lamb, and Deer Meat*

Please note: My comments below apply to all sorts of meat products sold in our stores: beef, pork, lamb, chicken, turkey, et cetera. Cook these meats exactly the same way you always do, just remember to avoid high heat, grilling and barbecuing, as these cooking methods will create toxic compounds.

Boeuf. *Beef*

I can just hear a sigh of relief coming from the meat eaters out there. The low-fat crowd wants you to believe that all meat is bad for you because it contains saturated fats. Well, there's meat and then there's meat. The kind I will tell you about is the healthier type of meat. How can meat be healthy for you?

First of all, meat contains nutritional elements hard to find anywhere else, such as vitamin B12 and iron in very easy to digest forms. After all, we humans are omnivores, meaning our dental structure and digestive system allows us to chew and digest a wide assortment of foods. While I understand there are vegetarians, vegans and raw-foodists in the world, and respect their opinion on what they choose to eat, I do not quite agree with them. Yes, we should eat a lot of vegetables but some of them need to be cooked to be edible or to unlock their health benefits. Yes, we can survive on vegetable, legumes, fruits, nuts and seeds alone but there is a good chance one can become B12 and iron deficient. Yes, I also understand that cooking some foods at high temperatures will kill all the beneficial enzymes, vitamins and minerals needed for our body to be and stay healthy, but cooking at low temperatures can help unlock the goodness hidden in many foods. So my personal belief is that we should eat a variety of foods prepared in different manners. Some raw, some barely cooked, some lightly cooked and some baked or boiled. As they say, variety is the spice of life and since I believe that good food should be enjoyed rather than be obsessed over, I endorse variety.

There is Meat, and there is Meat.

As I mentioned earlier in the Dairy section, the source of the meat we eat is very important. What you do not want to eat is the kind of meat that is raised in huge feedlots where the animals are crowded, mistreated, artificially "grown" with growth hormones, doused with pesticides and doped with antibiotics to keep them alive until they are "processed", cut up and wrapped under plastic film at your local supermarket.

Another thing to consider is the type of food these poor animals are fed. Since they cannot graze on pasture as it would take too much time, they are fed a diet of mostly grains, specifically corn. Corn maybe good roasted on the cob, but corn is not meant to feed animals, especially not cows. That's what makes their fat yellow and not white, as it should be. For one thing, their digestive system is not designed to digest corn. So it makes them sick to their stomachs and the side effect on our environment is methane. Additionally, corn provides an important source of omega-6 fatty acids that some scientists believe are inflammatory to our body. If you remember what I explained earlier, our diet should have an ideal omega-6 to omega-3 ratio of 3/1. In our modern diet, especially if you eat the SAD (Standard American Diet), your ratio is more likely to 15/1 and even all the way up to 25/3. That is potentially dangerous as it creates more degenerative diseases like heart disease and some forms of cancer. Why do you think we have such an increase in these diseases since the end of World War II? To paraphrase a famous political slogan, "It's the food, stupid!" Eat more food containing omega-3s (grass-fed meat and free-range eggs, cold water fatty fish, flaxseeds, chia seeds) and you will feel better.

The Other Red Meat: Grass-fed.

What you want to put in your body is (ideally) grass-fed meat coming from animals raised the way they should be, humanely and eating the kind of food they're supposed to eat: grass. You see, grass-fed meat contains more of the healthy fatty acids your body needs: omega-3 fatty acids and conjugated linoleic acid. Omega-3 fatty acids are not only good for your brain, they also keep your blood fluid by increasing your HDL (good) cholesterol and protecting you from oxidation and inflammation. So, if you can find it, buy and eat grass-fed meat.

Certified Organic Meat

Certified organic meat would be my second choice. Certified organic farmers treat their animals much better and do not use growth hormones, antibiotics and pesticides, but the organic feed they use is not fresh, green grass. It is usually composed of assorted grains (including corn), hay and even sometimes sea vegetables to add that extra omega-3 that would otherwise come from the grass. It is not bad by any means and is a much better choice than the "regular" meat. If you cannot find grass-fed meat, buy your meat certified organic.

Natural Beef

Unfortunately, "natural" is a marketing denomination opened to a very wide range of interpretations. Don't believe what some producers are trying to make you believe. If you can, stick with the above choices.

Shopping Budget Concerns

I do realize that for some people there is a financial factor involved. So, let me offer a suggestion. We do NOT have to eat meat every day, as the meat industry would like you to believe. Eating red meat once a week is plenty enough. You can also substitute white meat for red meat: chicken, turkey, or pork, if it makes it easier on the pocketbook. And we certainly do NOT have to eat a one-pound steak at every sitting. A 3-4 ounces serving per meal is plenty. I would much prefer you eat a smaller portion of better quality meat then a big chunk of "regular" meat. Please keep that in mind when you write your shopping list.

Alain's shopping advice

In Austin, look for **Always Grass-Fed Beef**, **Bastrop Cattle Company**, **Betsy Ross Farm**, **Dewberry Hills Farms**, **Richardson Farms**, and **White Egret Farm**. All are available at the local farmers' markets, from Greenling.com, and at several grocery stores.

Alain's Recipes: *Southern France Meat Loaf, page 215. Provencal-style Beef Stew, page 216.*

The Other, Other Red Meat: Bison or Buffalo

I know I seem to be veering dangerously off the French food here, but I thought I would mention this meat since it is a healthful meat that is increasingly accepted in the US. Also, there is a European Bison. They are currently raised in Eastern countries and even in France: I found a farm that raises European Bison in the Franche-Comte region called Les Bisons de Bacarat. There are efforts to reintroduce Bison into the wild again in Eastern Europe. The American Bison and the European Bison are not related, but are similar.

In the U.S., more and more farmers are raising grass-fed bison as a healthier alternative to beef. Since it feeds on grass, it contains the same health attributes as the grass-fed beef with its high omega-3 fatty acid content. It is also a leaner meat with more protein and less fat and calories per ounce.

Alain's shopping advice

In Texas, you can get bison from **Thunderheart Bison**, The **Bison Provision Company** and the **Lucky B Bison Ranch** sold at Whole Foods Market and Central Market, **Greenling.com** and at other local health stores.

Alain's cooking tips

Use the same techniques used to cook beef. Just remember that since their meat is lower in fat, you need to cook bison at lower temperatures and for less time, otherwise it will be tougher to eat.

Alain's Recipes: *Bison Cranberry Stew, page 218. Bison Roast with Hunters Sauce, page 220.*

Agneau. *Lamb*

I include lamb for two reasons. Firstly, for sentiment: I was raised Roman Catholic and in France, to celebrate Easter, we traditionally eat lamb with "flageolets", the tender green, melt-in-your mouth beans I mentioned in the beans section. The lamb we ate was special, raised in the pre-Alps region of Sisteron, on the Route Napoleon. For me, the thought of this meal always brings back happy memories. I also had the opportunity to eat lamb with couscous and cooked in a Moroccan tagine (a special cone-shaped dish used in Northern Africa to cook a moist, tender and flavorful meal.)

Secondly, because grass-fed lamb contains a good amount of omega-3 fatty acids, is low in fat and loaded with high-quality protein.

Alain's shopping advice

At the Austin farmer's market, for fresh lamb I suggest you look for **Loncito Lamb** and **Twin County Dorpers** or use Greenling.com. National brands can be found at **Central Market** and **Whole Foods Market**.

Alain's Recipes: *Provencal Lamb Stew with White Wine page 212. Lamb Filets Mignons with Sautéed Spinach and Spring Vegetables page 214.*

Chevreuil. *Venison*

I don't know about other states, but in Texas, hunters are allowed to shoot deer for sport or for eating. I'm not going to make any friends with the hunting folks here but I never quite understood the fun in killing defenseless animals for sport. I can appreciate the need for that when people used to depend on hunting to provide meat, but nowadays? A good friend of mine living in the Texas countryside, waits for the deer to "trespass" and shoots them right there on his property. Don't worry, it's all legal, and I have to admit he does make a mean deer "pâté" out the meat he dresses and cooks himself. To be honest with you, I must confess I have enjoyed his culinary results quite a few times over the years. Hypocrite? You're probably right. I guess you could say I bypass the guilt of eating deer by not killing it myself, just like most people do with beef.

We also have the same hunting traditions in France. The big difference is that they make a big show of it with people dressed in special hunting garb, horses and specially trained dogs. In this particular form of hunting, only the dogs do the killing and the humans are only there to control the dogs and prevent them from eating the deer. Well, you can tell by now I'm not a big fan of deer hunting in any form.

I include venison in the "meat" section only because, whether hunted or farm-raised, venison is a healthier meat than your average beef. It is much lower in fat and high in omega-3 fatty acids, since deer typically forage on wild grass and bushes. This can help lower your cholesterol levels.

Alain's shopping advice

After asking around, I finally found a ranch that provides humanely field-harvested venison, antelope and wild boar meat. Its name is **Broken Arrow Ranch** in Ingram, Texas. Otherwise, ask one of your hunters' friends. If you're nice, he may share some of its catch with you.

Alain's Recipes: *Deer Filet with Grand Veneur Sauce page 224. Deer in Cherry and Orange Sauce page 226.*

Cochon. *Pork* et Veau. *Veal*

Cochon. *Pork*

Pretty much the same thing I said for beef is applicable for pork. There is no such thing as grass-fed pork, but there is pork made from humanely raised pigs that have been fed good organic food. If possible try to buy pork meat that has not been cured with nitrates or nitrites. These are poisons to our body known to cause some forms of cancer.

Alain's shopping advice

In Austin, try **Richardson Farms** and **White Egret Farm, Peach Creek Farms** or **Greenling.com**. Otherwise, try **Applegate Farms** and **Organic Prairie** assorted pork products. Also look into your local **Central Market** and **Whole Foods Market** for national brands.

Alain's Recipes: *Grilled Pork Chops in Mustard and Sage, page 221. Baked Pork Chops with Apples and Cinnamon, page 222. Veal Chops with Côte d'Azur Pine Nuts, page 223.*

Volailles *Poultry* : Poulet *Chicken*, Dinde ou Dindon *Turkey*

Alain's shopping advice

For chicken and turkey, I recommend free-range, cage-free poultry, purchased directly from farmers, or from your local health food store. In Austin, look for **Barnison Farm**, **Country Grill Rotisserie Chicken**, **Dewberry Hills Farms**, **Richardson Farms**, and **White Egret Farm** at your favorite farmer' market, **Greenling.com** or health food store. Otherwise, look for **Organic Prairie** or similar in your neck of the wood.

Alain's Recipes: *Chicken Salad with Grapes and Toasted Walnuts, page 228. Lemon Herbs Roasted Chicken, page 229. Roasted Turkey with Prunes and Apples, page 230.*

Poissons et Fruits de Mer. *Fish and Seafood*

When I was still an apprentice in Nice, once in a while on Sunday (yes, we work on Sunday in the pastry business), to thank us for our hard work, the chef would treat us with "poutine". Poutine is a term used in Nice for tiny fish, usually sardines, too small to be prepared the usual way. They are dredged in flour and quickly fried like French fries and served hot in a newspaper cone sprinkled with sea salt and pepper. Think of them as a fish version of French fries. If you wish, you can dip them in mayonnaise, but not in Nice. There, we eat poutine "as is". Sometimes, it is prepared as a "beignet" (fritter). Since I was the youngest apprentice, some Sundays, I was sent out on my "mobylette" (moped) to the fish market to buy enough for all of us. What a treat! If you ever go to Nice, go to the fish market and ask for poutine. You won't be disappointed.

Fish and seafood are a very good source of high-quality protein at a low-calorie cost. They are my favorite source of protein. Possibly because coming from the Mediterranean part of France, we ate more fish than meat because fish was easier and cheaper to get. You could go to the local fish market and get fish freshly caught the same morning from the nearby sea. How could you beat that? Also, because Cote d'Azur is not a meat-producing part of France, fish was always more familiar to me. I eat an average of two to three servings of fish and seafood per week. I will not cover all fish and seafood; only the ones that can help us lower our cholesterol.

As in many other food sources, fish's quality depends on how and where it was caught or whether it was farmed or not. This is another subject that could become very complicated but I will try to keep it brief. If you are living near the sea or ocean, your first choice would be to pick fish harvested locally and delivered very quickly to your fishmonger. If you're not living close to the coast, I would suggest you find a local store that imports its fish daily or at least two to three times a week. In Austin, we're lucky to have a well-known fish wholesaler that also sells to the public and always has fresh fish available: Quality Seafood on Airport Boulevard. They supply the vast majority of seafood restaurants in town. Other good choices are Whole Foods Market and Central Market. Both of them have enough volume for you to know their fish is always fresh. If you're not sure, be sure to ask. I always ask my fish guy what arrived that day.

When it comes to fish and seafood, one of my pet peeves is that the health regulations are not nearly as consumer-friendly as they are for meat. That is another good reason to form a good relationship with your fish person. Once you get to know each other, he's more likely to tell you the origin of the fish you want to purchase. I hope the laws will improve in the near future; until then, educate yourself and ask a lot of questions.

Saumon. *Salmon*

Wild-caught Fish versus Farmed Fish?

Wild-caught
Here, I will make the same argument I did with meat. I'm going to use salmon as an example but the same reasoning applies to all edible fish. If you have the choice, go for wild, line-caught salmon first. I know it is more expensive, but I'd rather you eat 3-4 ounces of great fresh Alaskan salmon than 8 ounces of farm-raised salmon. For one thing, when eaten in season (yes, there is a season for catching salmon – August to October) nothing compares to fresh salmon in flavor, consistency and nutritional value.

On the nutritional side, there are two major reasons to choose wild salmon over farmed salmon. The first is that they are loaded with omega-3 fatty acids. And, if you remember my previous explanations on why omega-3 fatty acids are good for you, you already know they are extremely beneficial for your heart and brain health as well as increase your HDL (good) cholesterol. The other is that salmon, like some crustaceans (crayfish, shrimp, and lobster) are loaded with a powerful antioxidant called astaxanthin. It's a recently discovered antioxidant in the same family as beta-carotene and lutein. The red-orange pigment color wild salmon's flesh comes from eating krill, a tiny form of shrimp found in the ocean. They are loaded with this newly-discovered antioxidant. Some studies suggest that it is 100 times more effective as an antioxidant than vitamin E. Wow! Doesn't that makes you want to eat fresh salmon every day? As you may remember, antioxidants are needed to avoid the damage caused by the creation of free radicals. So the more antioxidants we eat, the healthier we will be. And fresh, wild-caught salmon is loaded with them.

If you're concerned with salmon's mercury content, salmon are too small to be contaminated with mercury when fished in season. They are not on the top of the food chain, so they do not accumulate this poisonous metal in their flesh. If you're pregnant or feeding a small child, you may want to be cautious, but for the vast majority of adults, two servings of fish per week are perfectly safe for you.

Farmed Salmon

As it is in the factory farms, so it is in fish farming. Their methods of raising fish are not a whole lot better for your health than feedlot methods are. Salmon (and catfish as well) are crowded in enclosures called "net-pens", which creates a potential for diseases to spread. So, the fish feed contains antibiotics to prevent that from happening. Since farmed salmon do not have the opportunity to eat their favorite food, krill, they are fed with artificially colored food pellets. If you pay attention at your fish market, you can tell farmed salmon from fresh as they have a weird, bright orange color.

Another thing you need to know is that farmed salmon are fed a grain diet, mostly made out of good old corn. Well, you already know the consequences of that. Salmon are carnivores. They eat other small fish to survive. That, in turn, will give them all the healthy attributes of a high amount of omega-3 fatty acids and the antioxidant called astaxanthin I mentioned before. What happens when they eat a grain diet is that their flesh now contains omega-6 fatty acids which are known to be oxidative and inflammatory to our body. So, not only you do not get the benefit of antioxidants, but also you are served an extra dose of inflammatory compounds.

If that wasn't bad enough, studies conducted by an independent group called the Environmental Working Group found that out of ten farm-raised salmon bought at grocery stores, seven were laced with a dangerous toxin: polychlorinated biphenils otherwise better known as PCBs. Since fish farms are located on or close to the coast, they are unfortunately polluted by toxic runoffs from rivers running into the ocean. To give you a comparison, farmed salmon contain sixteen times the amount of PCBs than in wild salmon. Doesn't that make you think twice about eating farmed salmon?

Alain's shopping advice

As I mentioned earlier, I have developed a good relationship with my fish person who keeps me updated on what's fresh that day. I buy small servings (4 ounces). Actually, in the beginning, my fish guy would tease me and ask me if I was buying fish for my cat. I laughed then told him I was on a special diet and left it at that. Now, when he sees me, he knows ¼ pound of fish is all I need.

Alain's cooking tips

I typically prepare my fish very simply and use short cooking times to preserve the unique flavor and health qualities of the fish I eat. I do not prepare complicated dishes because of the fact that I work in a kitchen all day long and don't have the energy to start all over when I get home. So I will give you quick and simple recipes for you to enjoy. Bon Appétit!

Alain's Recipes: *Alain's Quick Way to Prepare Salmon Filet, page 232.*

Sardines. *Sardines*

Their name come for the fact that, in ancient times, the Greeks noticed that sardines were abundant near the island of Sardinia in the Mediterranean sea. Being raised on the Mediterranean coast, I used to eat fresh sardines pretty regularly. Mostly, I ate them grilled, which is the way they are prepared in the South of France. But for the past years living in America, I had forgotten how good they are for one's health. That is until I read an article by one of my favorite doctors who believe in the healing power of food: Dr. David Williams. He was going on and on about the benefits of this fish, small in size but big in healthy attributes: canned sardines.

As you might guess, sardines are a great source of protein with many added benefits. Since you eat the whole fish (without the head), you receive a good amount of calcium from their bones. To make them more attractive to us, lower-cholesterol seekers, they are loaded with omega-3 fatty acids, the friendly omegas. Some people claim that they have the same amount of omeg-3 per serving as salmon, some say they're a close second. Either way, it's good news.

Alain's shopping advice

My favorite brand is a Portuguese brand called Bela Olhao. They come in plain and red peppers flavors. My other favorite brand is Crown Prince Wild Caught Brisling Sardines. They are both packed in pure olive oil. In Austin, you can find at Central Market and Whole Foods.

Alain's cooking tips

I first drain them of their olive oil (I give it to my cat. She loves it and it's great for her fur coat), spread them on my plate, drizzle them with lime juice and top them with a crush of sea salt and cayenne pepper. I always eat them with a side of mixed greens salad with my special homemade dressing.

Other not-to-be-forgotten fish and seafood

In my opinion, all fish and seafood are good, given the cautions I mentioned earlier: source and portion size. Crustaceans are some of the best for your cholesterol (crawfish, shrimp, lobster); they contain a good amount of the antioxidant I mentioned in the salmon paragraph: *astaxanthin*. Mackerel, a well respected fatty fish in Nordic countries, is a good choice; Mollusks (clams, oysters, scallops and mussels) are a good source of protein and zinc; Tuna – raw as in sushi or lightly grilled - is loaded with omega-3 fatty acids; and white fish such as cod, flounder, halibut, orange roughy, pollack and rockfish are good for you as well.

<u>**Alain's Recipes**</u>: Provencal-*style Mussels, page 233. Sea Bass in White Provencal Wine, page 234. Sea Bream with herbs cooked in Papillotte, page 235. Tuna Côte d'Azur-style, page 236. Trout Filets Amandine, p 238.*

Nourritures Spécialisées. *Specialty Foods*

Assortiment de Nourritures Fermentées. *Assorted Fermented Foods*

We need to go back to eating naturally fermented foods like sauerkraut, as they did in the old days, especially in Alsace Lorraine and of course Germany. Although I am not from Alsace Lorraine, since it is still in France, it qualifies for the purpose of this book.

I believe firmly in the benefits of fermented foods for our digestive system. Because I believe that our health starts in the gut, we need to keep it healthy by providing our bodies with live probiotics. Live probiotics are akin to the beautiful flowers found in your garden while other toxic bacteria and fungi like Candida are the weeds. To keep the weeds in check, you have to work at it and keep your flowers healthy. As in natural yogurts, naturally fermented foods contain lactobacilli. Fermented foods are known to support your digestive health, support your immune system and help control inflammation. Also keep in mind that the fermented foods mentioned in this paragraph are high in fiber.

Alain's shopping advice

A couple of years ago, the only fermented food I could find was miso. Recently, in Austin, there has been a resurgence of naturally fermented food producers. They are very small companies and only local. You can find their products at People's Pharmacy, Whole Foods Market and our local farmer's markets. If you look around in your area, you should be able to find similar products created locally. In German or Dutch parts of the country, it should not be difficult for you to find natural sauerkraut.

Alain's cooking tips

Sauerkraut can be eaten as a side dish at any meal. Try to avoid eating too many fat-heavy German sausages with it, though!

Poudre de Cacao Crue. *Raw Cocoa Powder*

Being a pastry chef for years, this is one product I'm particularly fond of. For the longest time in my career, I was not aware of this product's wonderful health attributes. I only discovered them after I became interested in nutrition. Now, be aware that all the following benefits come from natural cacao (not Dutch-processed cacao, a highly processed product) and better yet, if you can afford it, raw cacao powder.

Raw cocoa provides many beneficial compounds such as serotonin (an anti-stress neurotransmitter) and tryptophan (which fights depression). In our case, what piqued my interest is that raw cacao powder is high in flavonoids, powerful antioxidants as are found in red wine and green tea. The cocoa's special types of flavonoids are called *flavanols*. Flavanols are known to prevent the fat contained in our blood (cholesterol) from clumping together and creating clots or depositing as plaque.

Cocoa's polyphenol content has other benefits for us. It is believed to be more effective at cutting LDL (bad) cholesterol oxidation than red wine and green tea. It also contains magnesium, iron and calcium.

Alain's shopping advice

Now, I'm not telling you to go out and load up on sugar-loaded chocolate bars. What you should buy is high cocoa content chocolate bars; 70% should be the minimum. The rest should be real cocoa butter (not hydrogenated fats) and a little sugar (not high fructose corn syrup). The higher the cocoa content, the less sugar in it. In some European brands, you can buy it up to 92% but unless you like highly bitter food, I would not suggest it. I found my top limit to be 70%. That's also the type of chocolate I use in my desserts. European chocolate bars with high cocoa contents can now be found in most high-end grocery stores as well as health food stores. My favorites are the European brands such as Valrhona (France), Cacao Barry (France), Callebaut (Belgium), Lindt (Switzerland), and Valor (Spain). Good American brands are Guittard, Scharffen Berger, Dagoba, Vosges, and Ghirardelli. In Austin, you can find all or most of the above brands at Central Market and Whole Foods Market as well as other more specialized chocolate stores. The same can be said for other cities in the U.S.

As for cocoa powder, my favorite is Naked Organic Raw Cocoa powder, but there are plenty of other good brands. Try to find organic, raw cocoa powder processed at low temperatures, like olive oil. The low temperature protects its antioxidant benefits. In Austin, it can be found at People's Pharmacy, Whole Foods Market and Central Market. It should be available in most health food stores around the country.

Alain's cooking tips

My favorite morning drink nowadays is hot chocolate made with vanilla almond milk (you can use low-fat organic milk, soy milk, hemp milk or rice milk) blended with a half a teaspoon of raw cocoa powder (a little goes a long way) and local creamy honey. Be careful: raw cocoa is bitter. Adjust amounts to your taste. You can also add it to your morning smoothie if you wish.

My special treat in the evening is one (yes, only one) square of 70% dark chocolate. To enjoy it fully and make it last as long as possible. Let it melt on your tongue and linger there for as long as you can stand it. If you do it that way, you'll get all of the sinful flavors you want without the additional calories. I would like to warn some people: if you are a chocoholic, and cannot resist the appeal of chocolate, I would prefer you resist the urge. If you can stick to only one square, enjoy.

Alain's Recipes: *Cocoa and Almond Meringues, page 263.*

Boissons. *Beverages*

Although spring water is the best drink for hydration and a well-functioning body, it can be helpful to add a few other drinks for additional health benefits and variety.

Jus de Grenades. *Pomegranate Juice*

Did you know that in France, the same name is used for the fruit and the weapon? Originated from Southwest Asia, pomegranates can be found all over the Mediterranean basin. When I was young, my buddies and I would find the fruits, pry them open and share the seeds. We would suck the juice from the seeds, then spit them out as far as we could, like American kids do with watermelon seeds. I guess it's an international pastime for kids all over the world. We did not know then how healthy these little red seeds were, just that they tasted good and were a lot of fun to play with. I did not include them in the fruit section because, for most people, they are not worth the trouble to bother with. So, juice it is.

The most interesting part for us is that the flavonoids contained in these pomegranate seeds have two to three times the antioxidant power of red wine or green tea. That's a lot of antioxidant power and very helpful to prevent LDL cholesterol oxidation.

Alain's shopping advice

The best and easiest way to enjoy the health benefits of pomegranate is bottled juice. You may have noticed the plump, round bottles named **Pom**. Most grocery stores carry it. If not, check your nearest health food store.

Vin Rouge. *Red Wine*

This book not being a treatise on French wine, I will not get into the details of different regions, appellations and all that good stuff that wine aficionados relish. This liquid will only be addressed for its high cholesterol benefits.

You may have read or heard about the French paradox that has stumped scientists (especially in America) as they wonder (I will paraphrase here): "How is it possible for these French people, stuffing themselves with fatty foods like butter, cheese, cream and all sorts of decadent desserts, to have fewer heart attacks than Americans?" Some of them like to point their scientific fingers at red wine. It does not have to be French to work, but it seems to work better when French people drink French red wine. Just kidding! Nationalistic pride just kicked in. In my opinion, it's not fair to blame our dairy prowess for heart attacks.

As you know by now, I do not believe that saturated fat from dairy and animal products are the only culprits. I will admit that if you abuse them, it may have some influence. But the most recent discoveries point to the oxidation of these fats as the primary culprit in heart disease. If the animal fat is coming from grains, it will contain more omega-6 fatty acids, which are more prone to oxidation than the omega-3s. So our first goal, if possible, is to ingest more foods coming from grass-fed animals. But if that is too difficult to find, do as French do and drink up to two glasses (one for the ladies) of red wine (organic or unsulfured if possible) per day.

Grape skins contain a powerful antioxidant called resveratrol. Resveratrol is one of the most potent polyphenols found in grape skin and seeds. Red wine gets its color and antioxidant super powers from the grape skins and seeds pressed and fermented with the juice during the winemaking process. White wine also contains resveratrol, but in lesser amounts, as the grapes' skins and seeds are taken out earlier in the winemaking process. Some studies have found that red wine can raise HDL (good) cholesterol. Red wine also is suspected of helping to prevent blood from clotting and reducing damage done by oxidation to our blood vessels. On the other hand, too much alcohol can raise triglyceride levels, raise blood pressure and lead to weight increase. Please don't abuse this wonderful medicine; it works better in reasonable amounts.

Alain's shopping advice

As I am not a wine expert, I will not pretend to guide you into the "dédale" (labyrinth) of red wines, French or otherwise. Your local wine steward or wine salesman will be able to match your personal taste with your newfound interest in nutrition.

Alain's drinking suggestions

I believe that red wine should not be refrigerated; on the other hand, drinking red wine after your bottle has been sitting in the hot Texas sun may not be a good idea either. Just let the wine come back to room temperature before you serve it. This will allow its "bouquet" to flower the way it is intended to. Use the proper glass, and let your wine breathe before you savor it one sip at a time. Beyond this basic advice, you may want to ask someone more qualified than me in wine appreciation. I will share an ugly secret (for a Frenchman): all my life, I've relied on my wife or lady friends to pick the wine for me when dining out. There it is, out in the open. Oh well… nobody is perfect.

Alain's Recipes: *Red Wine Onion Soup, page 184. Prunes in red wine and cinnamon, page 261.*

Thé – vert, noir et blanc. *Green, Black and White Tea*

Originating in China, tea is one of the most ancient beverages known to man. It is the second most consumed beverage in the world. It is prepared differently in different countries:. in China and Japan, loose tea leaves are allowed to steep in hot but not boiling water for a few minutes then poured in delicate China tea cups and enjoyed straight; in England, it is steeped in a similar manner but usually enjoyed with a cloud of milk or a lemon slice, and perhaps a cube of sugar. In Mongolia, it is boiled for a long time with spices and served in pottery cups. Like most people, my mother used to drop a bag of tea in her cup and enjoy it with a cube of sugar and a lemon squeeze. Lately, tea has become the newest "hot" drink in the U.S. You can see tearooms sprouting all over the landscape. Since it is a healthy beverage, I can only applaud this new trend.

There are different denominations of tea depending on the way the tea leaves are processed. Without getting too complicated, since this is not a book about tea, the main tea choices are: White tea, Yellow tea, Green tea, Oolong tea, Black tea and post-fermented tea. For our purpose, the most important teas are the Green and Black teas. The progression is the result on how much oxidation the tea leaves have been exposed to.

For the sake of simplicity, green tea is not oxidized and black tea is fully oxidized. Green tea, being the least processed contains the most of one particular type of polyphenols called catechins, which are powerful antioxidants. Green tea has also been found to lower *fibrin*, a protein involved in blood clotting.

On the other hand, black tea is fully oxidized which eliminates the beneficial catechins. But during the fermentation process the black tea develops other forms of antioxidants called *biflavonols, thearubigens* and *theaflavins*. It turns out that theaflavins are as effective an antioxidant than catechins. In a recent research, these flavonoids helped reduce the production of LDL (bad) cholesterol. Theaflavins are also known to activate our own body's powerful antioxidant, SOD (superoxide dismutase). Black tea has also been shown to be superior to green tea in lowering triglycerides levels.

So pull out those fancy tea cups and enjoy your green or black tea any way you see fit and enjoy its positive effects on your cholesterol levels.

Alain's shopping advice

Since I am not a tea expert, I will not make a fool out of myself. I will only recommend that you find the nearest tea house and go talk to the owner. That person will know a lot more about tea than I will ever know.

Thé d'Hibiscus. *Hibiscus Tea*

This tea is brewed from the red hibiscus flower (***Hibiscus sabdariffa***) originally grown in the Nile Valley of Sudan and Egypt. It was known to be pharaohs' favorite cooling drink when they ventured into the desert. In countries as diverse as China, Mexico, Jamaica, and even Europe, hibiscus tea has been appreciated for centuries.

What makes this refreshing drink so special besides its beautiful color? For one thing, it is loaded with vitamin C, a known antioxidant. Hibiscus tea has also been found to help lower blood pressure. In an article in a 2009 issue of the Internal Medicine News, hibiscus tea is described as follows: "***Hibiscus*** *sabdariffa* has antihypertensive and antiatherosclerotic effects. Hibiscus contains flavonoids and phenolics acids that have potent antioxidant properties."

Another interesting finding is that hibiscus tea aids in the removal of triglycerides and cholesterol from blood vessels, which contribute to high blood pressure, blood clotting or blockage, and subsequent heart problems. So, there you have it, another healthy drink to help us lower our cholesterol levels.

Alain's shopping advice

In Austin, we are lucky to get our get our hibiscus tea from a local business called **Nile Valley Teas** (www.nilevalleyherbs.com). **Mr. Awad Abdelgadir**, a Sudan native, not only offers a wonderful product, he also uses part of the profits generated by his small business to help his home village get clean drinking water, a school, a clinic and other worthy projects. In Austin and surrounding areas, you can find Mr. Abdelgadir's hibiscus and hibiscus mint teas at local health food stores, restaurants, delis like **People's Pharmacy**, **Central Market** and **Whole Foods Market**, **Wheatsville Grocery**, **Fresh Plus** and many other Austin locations. Or, you can order directly from their web site.

Herbes et Epices. *Herbs and Spices*

Cannelle. *Cinnamon*

Who would have known? The humble spice everyone uses in their apple pie, pumpkin pie and many other dishes is also good for your health. Cinnamon has been revered since ancient times, as far back as the Old Testament where Moses commanded the use of sweet cinnamon and cassia in the holy anointing oil.

Cinnamon is known for its anti-inflammatory benefits and high antioxidant content. A recent study in *Diabetic Care* reported that in people with type 2 diabetes, cinnamon not only reduced blood sugar levels but more importantly for us, total cholesterol and LDL (bad) cholesterol as well as triglyceride levels.

Unlike some other plant extracts, the powder is more efficient in its healing power than the expensive oils.

Alain's shopping advice

The good news is that the cinnamon powder you can buy in bulk at your favorite store is the best and cheapest way to use it. If you can find it, Ceylan cinnamon is considered to be the finest variety, although less strong than the other form of cinnamon, cassia.

Alain's cooking tips

As anyone else in the pastry industry, I use it in a variety of desserts, even in my special Gluten-free Pumpkin Cheese Cake.

Gingembre. *Ginger*

In France, ginger is mostly used in "pain d'épices" (spice bread), otherwise known in this country as gingerbread, which originated in Alsace Lorraine. I used to love to get a slice of it covered with fresh butter for my afternoon "gouter" (snack) when I came home from school. That is only use I know of in France. It is used regularly in the Middle Eastern and Northern African countries.

In lab tests, ginger extracts inhibited the oxidation of LDL (bad) cholesterol and lowered total cholesterol levels.

Alain's shopping advices

I prefer to buy mine fresh, organic and young. When it gets too old, it becomes fibrous and bitter.

Alain's cooking tips

I use a good chunk of ginger in my home-made healthy salad dressing.

Alain's Recipe: *Alain's home-made healthy dressing p 251.*

Pantry staples

Breakfast Cereals: unsweetened muesli mix, steel-cut oatmeal, whole bran cereals, organic corn cereals.

Dried Fruits: If you can find them, buy bulk unsulfured fruits such as apricots, dates, and prunes.

Dried beans and rice: I have an assortment of dried beans, wild rice and organic brown rice in my pantry. I also have a few cans of canned beans for when I'm too tired or busy to cook beans from scratch.

Raw Nuts: If possible, buy them in bulk. They will be cheaper and fresher. Almonds (whole and sliced), walnuts (halves and pieces), pecans (halves and pieces), pistachios (not colored), pine nuts, macadamia nuts, cashews, Brazil nuts.

Seeds: Sesame seeds, pumpkin seeds, sunflower seeds, chia seeds, flaxseeds.

Whole Grain Crackers: Some of these contain dried fruits and seeds. They contain no yeast. I love them as a quick snack with nut butter, fruit preserves or cheese. Ryvita, Wasa, Dr. Cracker, Ak-Mak and Central Market Organic Crackers.

Canned products: Sardines, tuna in olive oil; organic beans: black, fava, garbanzo or others.

Tomato sauce: organic crushed tomatoes with basil. I use this to make my own easy tomato sauce with no added sweeteners. I sauté a small onion and 4 chopped garlic cloves in olive oil. Sprinkle sea salt and cayenne pepper. Add the can of tomatoes and simmer with a couple of pinches of the frozen herbs I mention below and/or some pesto sauce for additional flavor. Voila! You have a perfectly good homemade tomato sauce in about 5 minutes. Otherwise, there are plenty of very good quality organic tomato sauces out there, just skip the sugar.

Pasta: Speaking of which, I only use whole-wheat pasta. It is pretty easy to find these days. Avoid refined white pasta.

<u>Oils</u>: Extra virgin olive oil, macadamia nut oil (MacNut), extra virgin coconut oil (Spectrum or other brands).

<u>Vinegars</u>: I try to keep 2 or 3 flavors on hand for variety: my favorite is apple cider vinegar, then red wine vinegar and herbal vinegars.

<u>Mustard</u>: I only use Dijon mustard. There are a few very good brands in most grocery stores. Grey Poupon makes an acceptable substitute.

<u>Salt</u>: I use only sea salt. Coarse salt for cooking my pasta and for my oven-roasted rosemary potatoes. Fine for all other uses. The processed "regular" salt out there contain chemicals and has been overheated, which changes salt's molecular structure. Do not use it. Any good quality sea salt will do, whether it be from France, Italy or the Himalayas.

<u>Pepper</u>: I prefer to use cayenne pepper. It is also known to increase your basic metabolism and is reputed to be healthy for your stomach.

<u>Herbs</u>: When I don't have access to fresh herbs, I either use the trick below or use an assortment of organic herbs. My favorite is the Herbes de Provence blend from Central Market.

<u>Sweeteners</u>; I rarely use added sweeteners in my food. The only exception would be to sweeten my tea or coffee. On my kitchen counter, you will find turbinado (or sucanat) sugar, local honey and agave nectar. Nothing else. If you have blood sugar issues, you can use Stevia.

<u>Cocoa Powder</u>: I use Nestle or Hershey's unsweetened cocoa powder only. Do not buy the sweetened cocoa mixes; they are loaded with sugar.

<u>Chocolate bars</u>: I only eat dark chocolate with at least 70% cocoa content. If you can stand the bitterness, you can go up to 85%. Any of the good quality European or boutique American chocolate makers will do.

Refrigerator Staples

Dairy products

<u>Milk</u>: If possible fresh, non-homogenized, lightly pasteurized whole milk. If not, buy organic whole or skim milk. For people with lactose intolerance, use organic soy, almond, hazelnut, rice, or hemp milk.

<u>Butter</u>: If possible, raw butter. If not, organic cultured butter. I like French butter best, but there are good quality American butters available.

<u>Cheese</u>: I prefer my cheese local and unpasteurized. But I will not deny buying a good quality French cheese, even when it is pasteurized (that's the only way the U.S. government will allow any cheese to enter this country). I also have a weakness for goat cheese. Even if you are lactose intolerant, you should be able to digest cheese, as the fermentation and aging process eliminates the lactose. Please do not ever buy this waxy make-believe cheese they call American cheese, or the yellow stuff some people melt over their sandwich. There should be a law against calling these products cheese.

Meat and Eggs

<u>Beef</u>: If possible, grass-fed and local. If not, organic. Nothing else. Just buy smaller portions.

<u>Bison or Buffalo</u>: Since bison feed on grass, there should not be the same concerns as you have with regular beef. Just make sure they use antibiotics only when necessary and never use growth hormones. Ask your butcher.

<u>Lamb</u>: They are always grass fed and too young to be polluted with all sorts of chemicals. Just buy from a reputable source.

<u>Chicken and Turkey</u>: Buy organic if possible. Free range is a good choice if they are raised locally and you can actually check to see that they get a chance to roam free.

<u>Eggs</u>: If you know the farmer, by all means, free range is the best. Buy locally. Otherwise, organic and omega-3 eggs are a good choice.

<u>Seafood</u>: Buy line -caught fish in season if you can. Avoid farm-raised.

Fruits and Vegetables

<u>Fruits</u>: I always keep an assortment of seasonal fruit. If you can, buy locally. Next best is organic within your state. Then, organic out of state.

<u>Vegetables</u>: I always have a bag of organic mixed field greens in my refrigerator. I also have cherry tomatoes and avocados. Keep a variety of vegetables on hand according to what's available in season. Same shopping recommendations as for fruits.

<u>Caution</u>: If you cannot afford organic fruits and vegetables, you should know of the Dirty Dozen list of the most chemically sprayed fruits and vegetables. They are: Apples; Bell peppers; Cherries; Imported grapes; Nectarines; Peaches; Pears; Potatoes; Red raspberries; Spinach and Strawberries. They all have thin skins so more of the chemicals will seep into them.

<u>On the other hand, the least polluted fruits and vegetables are</u>: Asparagus; Avocados; Bananas; Broccoli; Cauliflower; Sweet corn; Kiwi; Mango; Onion; Papaya; Pineapple; Sweet peas. They are thick-skinned and are less likely to be chemically polluted.

<u>Nut butters</u>: My favorites are almond and hazelnut. If you can find them get the raw variety and keep it refrigerated as it will go rancid at room temperature within a couple of weeks.

<u>Fruit juices</u>: Honestly, I do not drink any bottled or boxed fruit "juices", as most of them are over-sweetened with high fructose corn syrup and contain only 10-15% of juice. Plus, they are pasteurized. All live vitamins and enzymes are dead. I prefer to drink water with a squeeze of lime juice in it. If you have the time, squeeze your own juice, or buy freshly squeezed juice at your local high quality grocery store like Whole Foods or Central Market. Just make sure they squeeze their own juices. Even in that case, I would suggest you cut that juice with equal amount of filtered water to reduce the sugar load.

<u>Water</u>: For me, the simplest and most economical solution is to buy a good quality countertop or under counter water filter and use that for drinking

and cooking. Fill up your stainless steel water bottle before you go to work and Voila! You're all set. No need to buy expensive bottled water unless it's a special treat like Perrier or Appolinaris.

Freezer Staples

Herbs: Here is a trick I learned during my last trip to France. To keep some fresh herbs "fresh" longer, pick or buy them fresh, take the leaves from the stems, chop them if you wish and store them in small freezer container with tight lids. They will keep that way for a long time and you will always have that fresh flavor available nearby. Rosemary and thyme are perfect examples. But some herbs with fragile leaves like basil will not survive the freezing process. A way to "save" them will be to make your own pesto sauce without the cheese in it and freeze it. Scoop it out as needed and its flavor will come alive in your dish.

Frozen fruits: I only eat fresh fruits, but frozen fruits can be useful for making smoothies. If possible, buy organic and unsweetened. Otherwise, stick to fresh.

Frozen vegetable: Same as above, fresh is always best. In special cases, organic flash frozen vegetables are preferable to conventionally grown fresh ones.

Ice cream: I would prefer you eat fruit sorbets or iced desserts made with coconut milk.

A Votre Santé and Bon Appétit!

Meal Recommendations

If you read nothing else in this book, the following section can function as a very abridged version. Please understand that this is not a diet, but rather suggestions put together in a somewhat organized fashion to help you get started. Here are a few main concepts to keep in mind, even if you don't follow this plan to the letter.

The No, No, Nos

- <u>Sugar is your enemy</u>: Pay attention to the amount of sugar you ingest in your daily diet. Avoid refined sugar in all its sneaky forms: white sugar, refined fructose, high fructose corn syrup, etc. Read the labels; sugar is added to nearly everything. Never eat artificial sugar.

- <u>Refined oils are not friendly either</u>: The vast majority of commercial oils have been damaged by heat through the refining process. They also possibly contain toxic compounds used to extract as much oil as possible. Do not touch the stuff.

- <u>Protein</u>: Your body really needs only 4-6 ounces of protein a day to stay healthy and rebuild itself. Anything over that amount is in excess and will tax your digestive system and kidneys.

- <u>Please do not obsess over this plan:</u> Take it one change at a time. Build up to it. I do realize that is it not always easy. I've done it for a long time and I still cheat once in a while. Just last night I ate a whole bag of fried veggie chips from my pantry. So be nice to yourself. Losing sleep over an occasional slip will not help.

The Yeah, Yeah, Yeahs

- <u>Sugar</u>: If you're going to use sugar anyway and have a choice, keep the overall amount low and use unrefined sugars (raw, turbinado, sucanat) or natural sugars like raw agave nectar, real maple syrup, or dark molasses.

- <u>Good fats</u>: When possible, use organic extra virgin olive oil, virgin coconut oil, macadamia oil and raw or organic cultured butter.

- <u>Dairy products</u>: Good quality dairy is acceptable in moderation: low-pasteurized, non-homogenized milk; raw or cultured organic butter; organic or natural (no sugar added) yogurt. Unpasteurized, locally-made cheeses are good for you, too. If you cannot have milk, soy milk (organic, non-gmo only), almond milk, rice milk, hazelnut milk, and hemp milk are all healthy alternatives.

- <u>Fresh Fruits and Vegetables</u>: Eat lots of fresh fruits and vegetables. They are loaded with beneficial fiber, vitamins, minerals and antioxidants. Eat 1 vegetable and 1 fruit at every meal. That should not be too difficult, even I can do that!

- <u>Eat a variety of proteins</u>: You do not have to eat meat every day. Once or twice a week is enough. Eat fresh fish or seafood at least twice a week. Nuts are also a good source of protein and healthy monounsaturated oils. Eat vegetable protein combinations like rice and beans, grains and pulse. Quinoa is another very good source of vegetable protein.

- <u>Food budget concerns</u>? To keep your food budget in line, keep portion size at a reasonable amount. Ideally, you should only eat the amount you could fit in the palm of your hand (rounded). Another good idea is to eat dinner leftovers for the next day's lunch.

- <u>Healthy gut beats leaky gut</u>: Keep your digestive system healthy with good quality fermented foods: plain natural yogurt and kefir, natural sauerkraut and kimchi, organic miso and tempeh (I know, they're not French, but since they're so good for you, I still recommend them.)

How to follow this meal plan

My first inclination was to give you a strict regimen to follow, but after some thought, I decided to treat you like adults and offer you guidance and suggestions instead.

To make it easier, I'm going to tell you how I do it. It's up to you to adapt it to your own use. It's your life, and I don't believe that dictating to you is going to help. These changes should not be a burden but a joy. Try to remember the French "Joie de Vivre" when you hit a snag. Good food is meant to be savored. Enjoy the process and try not to obsess about the final result. We both know you want to lower your cholesterol; enjoying the process will make it easier. If you are taking a cholesterol-lowering medicine, do not stop taking it before talking it over with your physician. Hopefully your doctor will be open to this diet-based approach.

I cook simple foods from scratch every day, quickly and with very little fuss. Many of the recipes in this book are for weekends and special occasions when you have plenty of time. The following ideas are my way of eating simply yet healthfully. Feel free to follow them or use them as an inspiration.

One of the main ideas I follow is the King, Prince and Pauper principle. Eat breakfast like a King, lunch like a Prince and Dinner like a Pauper. In other words, your best and richest meal should be breakfast, to charge you up for the day. Lunch should provide you with enough food to satisfy you, but not enough to put you to sleep at your desk. And dinner should be light so you do not overtax your digestive system before sleeping. Sleeping is for resting, not for digesting a heavy meal.

Breakfast

A normal French breakfast would consist of 2 tartines (pieces of French baguettes split in half) covered with either butter or fruit preserves, sometimes both, dipped in a bowl of "café au lait" (coffee with milk). Nothing else. In the old days, when I still lived on my grandparents' farm, the coffee was drunk very early in the morning (mostly by my grand-father before he did his early farm work) and then, when we kids woke up, we would have a more filling morning meal with eggs or some form of meat: ham, bacon or sausage. That would keep us going until lunch with no need for morning snacks.

Although when I go back home, I love to have my baguette and café au lait, with all due respect to my compatriots, this may not be the healthiest form of breakfast. I always complement mine with at least one egg for protein and a Muesli mix. In the recipe chapter, I give you my favorite breakfast cereal recipe and add a few easy egg dishes. For weekends, when you have a little more time, I added a few muffin and scones recipes, as well as recipes for wholesome pancakes and Pain Perdue (French toast).

Breakfast Sugar Alert
Excess sugar, in all its forms, is hidden in most of our modern breakfasts.

The sneaky product in most of our modern breakfasts is sugar in all its forms. Sweetened cereals, commercial fruit juices with added sweeteners, pancakes or waffles coated with imitation maple syrup and fruit toppings loaded with sweeteners. What's the problem with that kind of breakfast? All these refined flours and sweeteners may give you and your kids a boost for a couple of hours, but you will eventually experience a crash mid-morning caused by excess insulin. Too much blood sugar will also eventually raise your triglyceride levels, which leads to heart disease. So, feeling lethargic, you will naturally reach for your favorite sweet snack, coffee loaded with sugar or worse yet, a soft drink loaded with high fructose corn syrup. That may drag you through until lunch but this cycle is detrimental. If you keep on doing this for a long time, you will develop insulin resistance, which is your body's way of saying "I've had enough of these blood sugar ups and downs," and you will start to experience hypoglycemia and possibly Type II diabetes. Did you know that Type II diabetes used to be called Adult Onset Diabetes, typically caused by a lifetime of glycemic abuse? Nowadays, this condition is so prevalent in children that the name has been changed to Type II diabetes to differentiate it from Type I, the genetically-based kind. So I beg you, control the amount of refined sugars contained in your food and not only you will feel better but you will have more energy.

Kids and Sugar
Please keep in mind that children feel this blood sugar roller coaster more dramatically than adults. A lot of children are diagnosed as ADD/ADHD only because they cannot sustain attention in school when they experience the same mid-morning low you experience at the office. So they load themselves with soft drinks and the cycle intensifies. Many ADD/ADHD cases could be eliminated with a few simple changes to children's breakfast foods.

Alain's Breakfast Suggestions

<u>During the week and Saturday</u>: I eat my special healthy breakfast cereal (see recipe) with unsweetened vanilla almond milk, plain unsweetened yogurt, fish oil, flax or chia seeds and fresh fruits. Don't worry, there's plenty of natural sugar from the raisins and fruits to keep it sweet. You'll get lots of fiber, healthy oils from the nuts (monounsaturated) and the fish oil, or use flax seed oil if you can't stand the fish taste. You also get additional fiber and antioxidants from the fruits. I let this soak while I'm getting ready for work, then I add fresh fruits on top: half a banana or a few strawberries, blueberries, blackberries... whatever fruit is available in season. <u>Note</u>: you can use this same recipe blended for little kids. It makes a very tasty pudding-like confection.

I also have one egg poached in butter (see food recommendations), and a cup of warm chocolate almond milk. Don't use the premixed version, it's too sweet. Sugar is the first ingredient. Instead, make your own: buy the unsweetened vanilla almond or soy milk, add your own unsweetened cocoa powder, your sweetener of choice and blend before heating. Have a glass of lemon or lime water (1/2 lime squeezed in a glass of filtered water) to go with your medication or supplements. That's it. The variations come in the way you prepare your basic Muesli mix, the type of fruits you add and the way you cook your egg.

- <u>Sunday</u>: Usually, I prepare a French-style brunch: an omelet (see recipes), a mixed field green salad with my special vinaigrette (see recipe), a large bowl of cafe au lait, 2 toasted slices of country-style or sourdough bread spread with butter and a touch of Bonne Maman fruit preserves and finally, a fruit according to the season. You can't get more French than that.

Lunch

In smaller towns in France, most people still have a 2 to 3-hour lunch break. They go back home and eat a light meal, eaten with their family. Sometimes, they even have time to take a nap before going back to work (what a life!). In larger cities where the typical workday is 8 hours with a 1-hour lunch break, they do not have time to go back home, so many people bring a home-made meal in their lunch box.

Alain's Lunch Suggestions

I am lucky in that I have healthy food available at work. So I eat a salad with some protein on it (sliced ham, turkey or grilled chicken), with soup, whole wheat crackers, and fruit. During the week, it's easy for me because I have a whole deli at my disposal. I make a point of eating light since I do not have time for a nap and do not want to feel drained of energy from trying to digest a heavy lunch.

Salads: Typically, I alternate a healthy composed salad with a scoop of tuna salad or chicken salad on it. Sometimes I add a serving of natural oven-roasted ham or turkey breast with some Swiss cheese.

Sandwich: When I eat a sandwich, I use the French principle of "tartines", an open face sandwich with only one slice of bread. Or I order a half sandwich, which is enough for most appetites.

Soup: When the weather is cooler, I really enjoy eating our made-from-scratch daily soup with a couple of whole wheat crackers.

Other choices: Some days, I eat a serving of hummus, tabouleh, baba ganoush or beet salad with yogurt. A fresh fruit or a cup of fruit salad closes the meal. I avoid drinking water during my meals as it dilutes the gastric digestive juices. I do drink water during the day, just not during a meal.

Dessert: I know some people will disagree with this but I make a point of eating fruit at every meal. It's a very good source of soluble fiber and is loaded with fresh vitamins and minerals.

Lunch at work: If you have a cafeteria available at work, try to pick the healthiest items and avoid any fried food.

Fast food outlets: Of course, you already know that I'm not a big fan of fast food outlets (sorry, I refuse to call them restaurants as I feel it is an insult to real chefs trying to offer you real food.) If you don't have a choice, go ahead, but stick to the healthiest options. Avoid all fried food items (see chapter on fats) and stick with salads. One trick I use is to bring packets of healthier salad dressings and use that on my salad. Avoid their desserts; not only they are overly sweet, they most likely contain high fructose corn syrup (see the chapter on sweeteners).

Brown-bag it: Another way to eat a good lunch is to take healthy food you bought or made at home and pack it in a lunch box. It's a lot cheaper and you know exactly what went in that lunch. Pick foods listed in the "Foods Good For You" chapter, prepare them the healthy way and warm them up at work. Add a piece of fruit and you're all set.

Salads

In France, a salad is not considered a dish you serve before the main meal to make the guest wait while the main dish is prepared. It is either eaten after the main course or is the main course with an addition of some form of protein such as sautéed shrimps, grilled chicken, or nuts. A well-composed salad is a meal in itself. In the recipe section I provide you with a few salad recipes, both simple and complex.

I personally keep it very simple. When I do my shopping, I create my own mixed salad greens by picking an assortment of different greens and sprouts. I buy some cherry tomatoes, a few broccoli and cauliflower florets and a couple of avocados. When I get home, I mix my salad greens together, and place them in one of those green bags that will keep them fresh for a whole week. When I get home from a long day at work, I place a handful of mixed salad greens on a plate, add a few broccoli or cauliflower florets, a few cherry tomatoes, sometimes a sliced half of an avocado, and some nuts and drizzle on some salad dressing and Voila! A composed salad has been created. Sometimes I even add dried cranberries, raisins, sunflower or pumpkin seeds. Occasionally I may add a piece of grilled chicken breast or a broiled piece of salmon and I have a quick meal, 10 minutes tops. I save fancier salads for when I have special guests.

Snacks

When I was a kid, my mom would bring us our "goûter" as an after school snack. It mostly consisted of a piece of bread with a couple of squares of dark chocolate which in French is called "pain et chocolat". So some smart baker picked up on the idea and created the "pain au chocolat" (chocolate croissant). It is usually made with croissant dough wrapped around a bar of dark chocolate. Miam! (Yum!). Either way, it is a good and tasty way to fill the void between lunch and dinner. If you're lucky, you have access to a local bakery that offers chocolate croissants without having to go all the way to France. Otherwise, you may want to consider the healthy alternatives below.

- A fresh fruit, any fruit in season.
- Dried apricots with raw almonds.
- Pitless dates with walnut halves.
- Dried figs with pecan halves.
- Prunes with cubes of Swiss cheese. Trust me, it's very good.
- Baby carrots with ricotta cheese.
- Cream cheese with baby carrots, broccoli, cauliflower or celery sticks.
- Cottage cheese with berries or grapes.
- Mozzarella sticks with a small apple or pear.
- Dry-roasted peanuts with raisins.
- Plain yogurt sweetened with Stevia, agave nectar, honey or no-sugar added fruit preserves. Add high fiber cereals or oatmeal, fresh or dried fruits, sprinkled with ground fax seeds or Chia seeds.
- Swiss cheese cubes with fresh berries.
- Unsweetened applesauce with whole wheat crackers.
- Dried, crispy vegetable snacks with a fresh fruit.
- Corn, rice or vegetable chips with baba ganoush.
- Nitrate-free cold cuts with a slice of your favorite cheese.
- Toasted pita chips with hummus of your choice.
- Baked tortilla chips with bean spread or refried beans.
- Baked corn chips with guacamole dip and a touch of salsa.
- A slice of whole wheat bread with 2 squares of dark chocolate. Toast together in a toaster oven or toast the bread and let the chocolate melt on it. Yum!
- Whole-wheat crackers or whole wheat bread spread with your favorite nut butter and a touch of no sugar added fruit preserves.
- Whole-wheat crackers with a little organic mayonnaise and canned sardines or tuna.
- Whole-wheat crackers with a soft-boiled egg.
- Whole wheat crackers with Brie or Camembert cheese or any of your favorite local cheese.
- A slice of cold pizza (kidding, just making sure you're paying attention).

Fruit Smoothies

Smoothies are a good choice for a morning breakfast replacement or a healthy afternoon snack. If you make them at home, buy a bunch of bananas, let them ripen and slice them. Freeze them in one layer and pack them in a re-sealable bag. They are a perfect binder for smoothies, as they are loaded with fiber. Buy your favorite fruits pre-frozen so they are ready for use at a drop of a chef's hat. Have a container of soy or whey protein at hand as well. Fish oil and flax seed oil are good additions, too. As much as possible, if you cannot squeeze your own juice, use unsweetened or low sugar juices as bases for your smoothies. I personally love to use unsweetened vanilla almond milk as a base.

Recommended liquid bases: Coconut, soy, almond, hazelnut, rice, or hemp milk. Organic dairy milk. Unsweetened organic apple, orange and cranberry juices, or red wine (*kidding!*)

Recommended Fruits: frozen Acai fruit, organic bananas, peaches, mangoes, strawberries and raspberries.

Special juices: you can also add a shot of Genesis 4 Total Nutrition, Liquid Coral Calcium, Power 4 (Goji, Acai, Noni and Mangosteen juice), Noni concentrate, Mangosteen concentrate Goji Berry Concentrate, Acai concentrate, or Montmorency Tart Cherry Concentrate.

Protein powders: Soy, whey, or rice protein powder, or Metagenics UltraMeal.

Additional fiber: PaleoMeal fiber, Metagenics MetaFiber, Quantum Greens Mix, or Barlean's FortiFlax.

Cocoa powder: Sunfood Nutrition Raw Cocoa Powder.

Nut butters: Raw almond, Cashew, Coconut, Pecan, or Walnut butter.

Oils: Barlean's Fish Oil, Cod Liver Oil, Flax Seed Oil.

Supplements: Powdered Vitamin C, B and D3. Echinacea, Gingko, Ginseng, Daily Juice Power Source-C. Acidophilus.

This list should give plenty of options to play with. Enjoy!

If you happen to be in the neighborhood, your local Peoples Pharmacy can prepare the following specialty smoothies:

Antioxidant Smoothie: 10 oz Cranberry Nectar, 1 pack Sambazon Acai berries, 4 oz frozen Blueberries, 4 oz frozen Raspberries and 4 oz frozen Strawberries.

Probiotic Defense Smoothie: Probiogurt (goat yogurt fermented 30 hours), Acidophilus, Soy Milk, Frozen Mangoes and Raspberries.

Muscle Mania Protein Smoothie: Almond milk, Lecithin, Vitamin C, Whey Protein, Raw Almond Butter, Frozen Bananas.

Power Princess Protein Smoothie: Natural Apple juice, Flaxseed oil, fat-free vanilla Yogurt, Whey protein powder, and frozen Strawberries.

Sambazon Smoothie: Soy milk, Sambazon palmberry, Flaxseed oil, Ginseng, Mangoes.

Acai Energy Smoothie: Apple or orange juice, frozen Acai berry, Guarana, frozen Bananas, frozen Raspberries.

Acai Power Protein Smoothie: Apple or orange juice, frozen Acai berries, Guarana, soy or whey protein powder, frozen Bananas, frozen Strawberries.

Amazon Superfood Smoothie: Apple or orange juice, frozen Acai berries, Guarana, Super Green Formula, frozen Bananas, and frozen Strawberries.

Amazon Cherry Smoothie: Orange juice, frozen Amazon Cherry, frozen Strawberries.

Amazon Immunity: Vanilla soy milk, frozen Amazon Cherry, Ginger, Echinacea, frozen bananas.

And many others, according to season. Come by and let us make one for you.

Dinner

Ideally, this is a family meal. These days, especially when you have kids, outside activities are taking a toll on dinners eaten with the family in a quiet environment. If at all possible, try to have at least a few meals at home per week with no interruptions. You probably think I'm dreaming, but I do believe that in the long run, it will benefit the whole family's health, physical and mental. Because I know modern parents are busier than ever, so I will provide you with quick and simple ideas so you can prepare a meal in less than 30 minutes. I will also give you a few more fancier recipes for when you have a little more time on the weekend.

Alain's Dinner Suggestions

If you can, you should have a protein, a side dish and some fruit at every meal.

Soup and Salad: I love soups and I love salads. In cold weather, I would eat a bowl of soup with some protein in it (beef, chicken or fish), a salad and a fruit. This way, I have 50% of my meal raw (salad and fruit) and 50% cooked (soup with protein). In Summer, I eat a small portion of protein (meat, fish, egg) with a salad and a fruit.

Protein: You can prepare a quickly broiled small portion (4-6 ounces) of protein (grass-fed beef, organic chicken, turkey or fish), a salad with my special salad dressing (see recipe) and a fruit.

Eat Light at Night: What people don't realize is that we do not need to eat heavy meals at night just because that's when we have more time to eat. Our body functions a lot better and feels a lot lighter when you leave the table satisfied, but not stuffed. I also recommend you eat your last meal of the day at least 3 hours before going to bed. This way, your body will have enough time to digest your food before you go to rest, and you will sleep better and not gain weight.

Carbohydrates: If you can, avoid eating a large amount of carbohydrates at night. Because your digestive system slows down at night and you do not typically go through physical exertion, you body will tend to store carbohydrates at night more than during the day. Of course, if you plan to go out and dance all night, that rule may be ignored.

<u>Drinks</u>: If you need help going to sleep, you should drink a calming herbal tea like chamomile or warm milk or read a boring book. They all work for extremely well for me.

<u>Red Wine and Dark Chocolate</u>: Most evenings, I would end my dinner with a glass of red wine and, as a special treat, one (yes, I mean one) square of dark chocolate (70% cocoa content minimum).

Desserts

Unlike what you might think while strolling on a typical French street lined with fancy pastry shops, French natives do not eat a lot of pastries. They eat fruit. Pastries are usually reserved for a special occasion like a birthday or for a special guest at dinner. Sometimes, in a bourgeois family, they might purchase a box of "patisseries" for their Sunday brunch, always eaten at home. Sweets are also enjoyed with a friend (or friends) around a cup of tea or beverage in the afternoon.

I would like to tantalize your sweet palate with a few classic desserts as well as wholesome fruit desserts. Unlike American cakes, French desserts and pastries are light on sugar and complex in flavors. We do not like the sugar flavor to overwhelm the other ingredients. I always told my pastry students that a well designed cake or dessert is like a symphony. You must compose it with assorted ingredients whose flavors work well and compliment each other without any one overpowering the other. It is true that in some cases, one ingredient is the star of the show, like in a chocolate mousse. Although the main ingredient is chocolate, you do not want the mousse to be overly strong or too sweet. A "dessert réussi" (successful dessert) is a delicate balance of flavors that play happily with each other. Enjoy yourself without guilt! One good dessert a week will not kill you (really!) as long as you eat fruit for the rest of the week.

Alain's Dessert Suggestions
On a daily basis, focus on a variety of fresh fruits for breakfast, lunch and dinner. On weekends and special occasions, by all means enjoy a fabulous dessert, but keep in mind that most typical American desserts are loaded with refined flour, sugar and hydrogenated fats.

<u>Cakes</u>: If you can, make your own desserts from scratch with good quality ingredients and a low amount of sugar. I you don't have the time or skills, there are enough high quality bakeries in Austin to help you with a good cake or dessert. I would suggest **Sweetish Hill Bakery**, **Texas French Bread**, **Whole Foods Market** and the **Central Market** pastry counters. The pastries offered now are head and shoulders above what was available when I started my own French Bakery and Café in 1988.

<u>Frozen Desserts</u>: Instead of ice cream, which is typically loaded with refined sugar or high fructose corn syrup, I would suggest you look at fruit sorbets sweetened with raw sugar or agave nectar, or frozen desserts made with coconut milk, such as **NadaMoo** and **Coconut Bliss**.

One Week Meal Plan

To help you get started, I offer you some suggestions below and from then on, feel free to create your own menu based on the food ideas and recipes in this book. Bonne Appétit!

Monday

<u>Breakfast</u>: A Votre Santé Home-made Breakfast Cereal **(see recipe)** with milk (or alternative milk), chia or flax seeds, fish or flax seed oil, 1 Tbsp plain yogurt and ½ a banana sliced or a few berries; 1 or 2 eggs poached or gently cooked in butter; 1 glass of lemon or lime water; 1 cup of hot chocolate, coffee or café au lait.

<u>Lunch</u>: A small salad with your dressing of choice; one scoop tuna salad or a can of sardines in olive oil; 1 slice of whole wheat or grain bread; 1 apple; 1 glass lemon or lime water or iced tea, lightly sweetened.

<u>Afternoon Snack</u>: Dried apricots with raw almonds

<u>Dinner</u>: A 4 ounce grass-fed ground beef patty with Dijon mustard; small mixed field green salad with cherry tomatoes and sliced almonds with Alain's Healthy Dressing (see recipe) or your dressing of choice; 1 grapefruit; 1 glass of red wine and a square of dark chocolate.

Tuesday

Breakfast: A Votre Santé Home-made Breakfast Cereal (see recipe) with milk (or alternative milk), chia or flax seeds, fish or flax seed oil, 1 Tbsp plain yogurt and ½ a banana sliced or a few berries; 1 or 2 eggs poached or gently cooked in butter; 1 glass of lemon or lime water; 1 cup of hot chocolate, coffee or café au lait.

Lunch: A cup of People's Pharmacy hummus (see recipe) with 4 whole-wheat crackers; 1 slice of whole wheat or grain bread; 1 peach; 1 glass lemon or lime water or iced tea, lightly sweetened.

Afternoon Snack: Prunes and cubes of Swiss cheese.

Dinner: A 4-ounce sole filet sautéed in butter with sliced almonds (see Trout Filet Amandine recipe); Mixed Field Green Salad with Concord Pear, Walnuts and Roquefort (see recipe); 1 apple; 1 glass of red wine and a square of dark chocolate.

Wednesday

Breakfast: A Votre Santé Home-made Breakfast Cereal (see recipe) with milk (or alternative milk), chia or flax seeds, fish or flax seed oil, 1 Tbsp plain yogurt and ½ a banana sliced or a few berries; 1 or 2 eggs poached or gently cooked in butter; 1 glass of lemon or lime water; 1 cup of hot chocolate, coffee or café au lait.

Lunch: A small salad with your dressing of choice; one scoop chicken (see Chicken Salad with Grapes and Toasted Walnuts recipe); 1 slice of whole wheat or grain bread; 1 banana; 1 glass lemon or lime water or iced tea, lightly sweetened.

Afternoon Snack: Whole-wheat crackers or whole wheat bread spread with your favorite nut butter and a touch of no sugar added fruit preserves.

Dinner: 2 slices of untreated oven-roasted turkey breast with Dijon mustard; Baby Spinach Salad with Raspberries and Almonds (see recipe); ½ melon; 1 glass of red wine and a square of dark chocolate.

Thursday

Breakfast: A Votre Santé Home-made Breakfast Cereal (see recipe) with milk (or alternative milk), chia or flax seeds, fish or flax seed oil, 1 Tbsp plain yogurt and ½ a banana sliced or a few berries; 1 or 2 eggs poached or gently cooked in butter; 1 glass of lemon or lime water; 1 cup of hot chocolate, coffee or café au lait.

Lunch: A small salad with your dressing of choice; Two slices of untreated oven-roasted turkey or Black Forest ham with Dijon mustard; 1 slice of whole-wheat or other whole grain bread; 2 plums; 1 glass lemon or lime water or iced tea, lightly sweetened.

Afternoon Snack: Baked corn chips with guacamole dip and a touch of salsa.

Dinner: 1 pint Traditional Du Puy Lentil Soup (see recipe); 1 slice whole-wheat or other whole grain bread; small mixed field salad with 1 sliced tomato and sunflower seeds with Alain's Healthy Dressing (see recipe) or your dressing of choice; 6 strawberries; 1 glass of red wine and a square of dark chocolate.

Friday

Breakfast: A Votre Santé Home-made Breakfast Cereal (see recipe) with milk (or alternative milk), chia or flax seeds, fish or flax seed oil, 1 Tbsp plain yogurt and ½ a banana sliced or a few berries; 1 or 2 eggs poached or gently cooked in butter; 1 glass of lemon or lime water; 1 cup of hot chocolate, coffee or café au lait.

Lunch: A small salad with dressing of choice; 1 cup Traditional Du Puy Lentil Soup (see recipe); 1 slice of whole wheat or grain bread; 1 orange; 1 glass lemon or lime water or iced tea, lightly sweetened.

Afternoon Snack: Whole-wheat crackers with a soft-boiled egg.

Dinner: 4 ounces oven-roasted chicken breast with herbs (see recipe for Lemon and Herb Roasted Chicken); 1 slice of whole-wheat or other whole grain bread; Mixed Field Greens with Concord Pear, Walnuts, and Roquefort (see recipe); small bunch of grapes; 1 glass of red wine and a square of dark chocolate.

Saturday

Brunch: 1 cup of hot chocolate, coffee or café au lait ; 2 egg potato omelet with herbs (see recipe); small mixed field greens salad with your dressing of choice; Raspberry Muffins (see recipe); 1 glass of lemon or lime water.

Afternoon Snack: Dried figs with pecan halves.

Dinner: Soupe a l'Oignon au Vin Rouge (see recipe); Lamb Chops with Sundried Tomato Butter (see recipe); Radicchio, Blood Orange, Arugula and Olive Salad (see recipe); Peach sorbet (see recipe); 1 glass of red wine and a square of dark chocolate.

Sunday

Brunch: 1 cup of hot chocolate, coffee or café au lait ; Fines Herbs Omelet with Goat Cheese (see recipe); small mixed field greens salad with your dressing of choice; My "Mamie's" French Toasts (see recipe); 1 glass of lemon or lime water.

Afternoon Snack: A slice of whole wheat bread with 2 squares of dark chocolate. Toast together in a toaster oven or toast the bread and let the chocolate melt on it.

Dinner: Sea Bass in White Provencal Wine (see recipe); Asparagus, Garden Herbs and Parmesan Salad (see recipe); Light as Cloud Raspberry Soufflé (see recipe); 1 glass of red wine and a square of dark chocolate.

Recettes. *Recipes*

Petit Dejeuner. *Breakfast*

Petits Gâteaux à la Poêle aux Bleuets et Noix de Pecan.
Blueberry Pecan Pancakes

This is not really a French recipe but if you'll allow me, we'll call it a French Canadian recipe. I wanted to include it to give you a recipe with nut fiber and oil, as well as fiber and antioxidants from the blueberries. Voila!

Servings: 4

PROCEDURE

Prep Time: 15 min.

Cooking Time: 20 min.

INGREDIENTS

- 2 cups organic whole wheat pastry flour
- ¼ tsp sea salt
- 2 ½ tsp baking powder
- ½ cup pecan pieces
- 1 cup milk or unsweetened soy/almond/hemp milk
- 1 Tbsp apple cider vinegar
- ½ cup water
- 2 tsp extra virgin olive oil, for the pancake batter
- 1 cup blueberries, fresh or frozen
- 1 oz melted butter

- Mix all the dry ingredients, including the pecan pieces, together in a large bowl.
- In a separate bowl, combine the milk, vinegar and olive oil. Allow to set for 10 minutes, turning it into buttermilk. Combine the water with the rest of the liquids.
- Whisk the wet ingredients in with the dry.
- Fold in the blueberries carefully.
- Heat and butter a pancake griddle or cast iron skillet.
- Ladle 1/3 to 1/2 cup batter for each pancake onto the griddle.
- Fry until golden at the edges and the top starts to form bubbles.
- Flip over and fry until golden.
- Remove and place on a serving plate.
- Repeat until all batter is used.
- Serve with butter and pure maple syrup, unsweetened applesauce, or sugar-free fruit preserves.

Muffins aux Framboises. *Raspberry Muffins*

I love raspberries. They bring you a good dose of fiber and antioxidants. Feel free to use organic frozen raspberries if they are out of season. If you want to go nuts, add chopped almonds.

Servings: 4

Yield: 8 muffins

Prep Time: 20 min.

Cooking Time: 20 min.

INGREDIENTS

- 1 ½ cup whole wheat pastry flour
- 1 ½ tsp baking powder
- ½ tsp salt
- 1 ½ Tbsp raw sugar
- 1 egg, beaten
- 1 cup cold milk
- 4 Tbsp melted butter
- ¾ cup fresh or frozen raspberries
- ¼ cup almonds, chopped

PROCEDURE

- Preheat oven to 350° F.
- Mix dry ingredients together in a medium size bowl.
- In a small bowl, blend egg, milk, and butter.
- Add to the dry ingredients and mix just until lumpy.
- Add raspberries, stirring gently. Do not over mix.
- Spoon into greased muffin tins.
- Bake for 25-30 minutes or until a knife's blade comes out clean.
- Let rest for about 10 minutes. Take out of the pan. Eat warm.
- Chef's tip: This recipe is using what is called the muffin mixing method. Mix the dry ingredients in one bowl. Mix the wet ingredients in another bowl. Add wet into dry, mix gently and quickly and fold in the fruits and nuts gently at the end.

Biscuits aux Canneberges et Noix. *Cranberry Scones and Walnut Pieces*
You might think scones are an English creation…and they are. But I came up with my own version. Try it; it's so good, you might even think it's French.

Servings: 4

Prep Time: 15 min.

Cooking Time: 20 min.

INGREDIENTS

- **1 cup whole wheat pastry flour**
- **1 ½ Tbsp raw sugar, plus more for sprinkling tops**
- **½ Tbs baking powder**
- **3/8 tsp sea salt**
- **3 oz butter, cold, cut into pieces (3/4 stick)**
- **¾ cup fresh cranberries (or blueberries), picked over and rinsed**
- **½ tsp grated lemon zest**
- **½ cup walnut pieces**
- **3 Tbsp heavy cream, plus more for brushing tops**
- **1 large egg, lightly beaten**

PROCEDURE

- Adjust rack to center of oven, and heat to 400°F.

- Place a sheet of parchment paper on a baking sheet, and set aside.

- In a large bowl, sift together flour, sugar, baking powder, and salt.

- Using a pastry blender, or two knives, cut in butter until the largest pieces are the size of small peas.

- Stir in blueberries, zest and walnut pieces.

- Using a fork, whisk together the cream and the eggs in a liquid measuring cup.

- Make a well in the center of the dry ingredients, and pour in cream mixture.

- Stir lightly with your fingers just until dough comes together. Knead a few times to mix well. Do not over mix.

- Using an ice cream scoop size of your choice, scoop out dough onto the prepared baking pan.

- Pat them lightly. Brush tops with cream, and sprinkle with sugar.

- Bake until golden brown, 20 to 22 minutes.

- Transfer scones from baking sheet to wire racks to cool.

✓ Chef's tip: If the fresh cranberry season is over, this recipe works well with dried cranberries.

Muffins Fondants aux Noix. *Tender Walnut Muffins*

This recipe is a little rich, so reserve it for a special occasion. It is loaded with good fiber and you're getting a nice serving of omega-3s from the walnuts.

Servings: 6

Yield: 8 muffins

Prep Time: 15 min.

Cooking Time: 20 min.

INGREDIENTS

- **4 Tbsp butter, melted**
- **2 Tbsp honey**
- **2 eggs**
- **1 cup sour cream**
- **2 cups whole wheat pastry flour**
- **1 tsp baking powder**
- **1 pinch sea salt**
- **1 cup walnut pieces (other nuts (pecan, almond, hazelnut, pine nut) plus...**
- **1/3 cup walnut pieces for topping**

PROCEDURE

- Preheat oven to 350˚F.
- In a large mixing bowl, mix the melted butter with the honey, eggs and sour cream until well blended.
- Sift the flour, baking powder and salt over the creamed batter. Mix well and gently. Do not over mix.
- Fold in the nuts.
- Drop into buttered muffins tins (or sprayed with oil spray).
- Top with additional walnut pieces.
- Bake about 20 minutes until a small knife's blade comes out clean.
- Let cool 10 minutes in the pan. Take out of the pan.
- Serve warm with your favorite sugar-free fruit preserves.

- <u>Chef's tip</u>: The trick here is to not over mix this batter as it will strengthen the gluten and make your muffins tough and dry. Quick and gentle is the ticket.

Petit Déjeuner A Votre Santé. *A Votre Santé Healthy Home-made Breakfast Cereal*

This recipe is one I created for myself, based on the work of Dr. Budwig of Germany. It is low in sugar, full of soluble fiber and beneficial omega-3 fatty acids. The organic whole milk yogurt will provide live probiotics as well. When you choose to use the buckwheat cereal, it also makes it wheat/gluten-free.

Servings: about 30

Prep Time: 10 min.

Finishing Time:

20 min.

INGREDIENTS

To Start:

- **1 box of unsweetened Swiss Muesli Mix (Familia)**

- **OR Maple Glazed Buckwheat Flakes (Nature's Path)**

- **OR 1 lb organic, unsweetened bulk Muesli mix of choice**

PROCEDURE

- In a large bowl, mix the cereals with the fruits and nuts.

- Place in a glass or metal storage container with a tight lid.

- When ready to use, measure 1/2 to 1cup of healthy cereal mix into a bowl.

- Add the ground flax seeds or whole chia seeds (good for omega-3 fatty acids and good fiber for digestion).

- Pour 1 to 2 ounces of milk of your choice.

- Add 1 heaping Tbsp of yogurt.

- Top it off with 1 Tbsp of Fish, Cod Liver or Flaxseed oil.

- Mix well. Let it sit for 10 minutes to let the cereal absorb the liquids.

✓ Chef's tip: In Winter, I let my breakfast warm up at 200F in my toaster oven for another 10 minutes while I get ready for work.

- 1 cup sliced raw almonds
- 1 cup raw walnut or pecan pieces
- 1 cup raw sunflower seeds
- 1 cup raw pumpkin seeds
- 2 cups raisins or currant or dried blueberries
- 1 cup candied ginger

Before eating:

- 2 tsp flax seeds (ground) or chia seeds (whole)
- 2 oz soy, almond, hemp, hazelnut, or rice milk (your choice)
- 3 tsp unsweetened organic yogurt or soy yogurt (Whole Soy)
- 1 Tbs Fish oil, Cod Liver oil or Flaxseed oil

Pain Perdu de ma Grand-mère. *My "Mamie's" French Toast*

The way my grand-mother taught me, French toast is not a fancy dish the way it is perceived in America. It's only a poor folks way to rescue stale bread that's too hard to eat. In French, "pain perdu" means lost bread. So, in order not to waste precious bread, someone came up with this tasty way to rescue the lost bread. It is best done with stale "pain de campagne" or country style whole wheat bread, but you can try other breads. I hear making it with stale Challah bread gives great results.

Servings: 6

Yield: 12 slices

Prep Time: 10 min.

Cooking Time: 15 min.

INGREDIENTS

- **1 cup whole milk (or soy or almond or hemp milk)**
- **4 Tbs raw sugar**
- **½ tsp vanilla extract**
- **5 eggs**
- **1 pinch sea salt**
- **4 Tbsp butter or ghee**
- **12 slices of stale country style whole wheat bread (or brioche or challah bread)**

PROCEDURE

- Mix the milk with the sugar and vanilla extract, and warm to body temperature.
- When the sugar has dissolved, pour into a shallow dish.
- In another shallow dish, beat the eggs and salt as you would for an omelet.
- Add a pat of butter (or ghee, clarified butter) to your frying pan. When it sizzles...
- Dip each bread slice into the milk, back and forth. Do not allow to soak.
- Then do the same in the egg mix.
- Place in your frying pan. Add as many bread slices as your pan will accept comfortably.
- Cook on the first side for about 1 minute until golden.
- Flip carefully. Cook the other side.
- When done, reserve on a plate covered with a clean "torchon" (kitchen towel) folded over the toast to keep them warm.
- If you wish, you can sprinkle a little powdered sugar on top, or use your favorite topping: fruit preserves, honey, etc. I like mine with raspberry preserves.

Plats aux Oeufs. *Egg Dishes*

Omelette aux Pommes de Terre à la Manière d'Alain. *Alain's Way of making a Potato Omelet*

In France, we do not add milk or cream to our eggs when making an omelet. We also like our omelets "baveuses" (runny). I know, gross! But that's the way they taste the best! Give it a try; you may like it.

Servings: 4

Prep Time: 10 min.

Cooking Time: 10 min.

INGREDIENTS

- **2 Tbsp extra virgin olive oil or coconut oil**
- **2 Tbsp butter**
- **2 medium Yukon Gold potatoes, sliced thin**
- **8 eggs**
- **½ tsp sea salt**
- **¼ tsp cayenne pepper**
- **Fresh parsley chopped for decoration**

PROCEDURE

- The secret of a good omelet is that all your ingredients must be at room temperature, especially your eggs.
- Beat your eggs with the sea salt and cayenne (once in a while, I like to add some Provencal herbs to it for added flavor). The salt will break down the eggs albumin and make the omelet creamier (without adding cream).
- Slice your potatoes thin but not too thin (about 1/8th of an inch for the engineers out there).
- In a large frying pan on medium heat, melt the butter with olive or coconut oil. When the fat is hot but not smoking, place your potato slices carefully at the bottom of the pan. Cook on each side until golden.
- Just at the time your potatoes are done, turn off the heat and pour the eggs all over the potatoes. With a heat-proof rubber spatula, stir your omelet carefully until it's almost set. Transfer immediately to the serving platter.

Omelette aux Fines Herbes et Fromage de Chèvre. *Fines Herbs Omelet with Goat Cheese*

This is a lively omelet filled with the flavor of fresh herbs and the slight saltiness of fresh goat cheese. A lovely dish for a family weekend brunch.

Servings: 4

Prep Time: 10 min.

Cooking Time: 10 min.

INGREDIENTS

- **8 large eggs**
- **1 Tbsp fresh chives, chopped fine**
- **1 Tbsp fresh parsley, chopped fine**
- **1 Tbsp fresh chervil, chopped fine**
- **1 Tbsp fresh rosemary, chopped fine**
- **½ tsp sea salt**
- **½ tsp cayenne pepper**
- **2 Tbsp extra virgin olive oil or coconut oil**
- **2 Tbsp butter**
- **8 Tbsp fresh goat cheese, crumbled**

PROCEDURE

- Remember, all ingredients must be at room temperature.
- Chop your fresh herbs. Beat the eggs; add the herbs, salt and cayenne. Mix well. Let sit for 5 minutes to allow the salt to softened the eggs.
- Heat your frying pan at medium high heat; melt the butter and oil; when the butter fizzles, pour your eggs in the pan. Stir gently with a heat-proof rubber spatula.
- When it barely starts to set, crumble the goat cheese all over it and fold in half. Slide on the serving platter immediately.

✓ Chef's tip: The goat cheese will melt inside your omelet and give you a creamy salty center. Yum!

Hors d'Oeuvres. *Appetizers*

Tapenade. *Tapenade*

This is a wonderful appetizer loaded with black olives and a touch of capers. Its original name comes from a loose translation of the Provencal word "tapeno" which means "capers". In my modest opinion, they should have called it "olivado" since there are many more olives. Go figure!

Servings: 4

Prep Time: 30 min.

INGREDIENTS

- **1 garlic clove, chopped fine**
- **2 Tbsp capers, drained and chopped fine**

- **8 oz pitted black olives Niçoises**
- **¼ tsp freshly ground black pepper**
- **8 anchovies filets in oil, drained**

- **8 to 10 Tbsp extra virgin olive oil**

- **One French baguette, sliced and toasted**

PROCEDURE

- Chop the capers and garlic finely with a chef's knife.

- Place the olives in the bowl of a food processor fitted with the metal blade. Chop by pulsing until coarse.

- Add the chopped garlic and capers, pepper and anchovies. Pulse until finely chopped.

- Add the olive oil and incorporate with a few additional pulses.

- Toast your French bread slices lightly. To enjoy, top each slice with tapenade and munch with delight.

✓ <u>Chef's tip</u>: Please do not over-process. This should not be a cream or a paste. It tastes a lot better if you leave it kind of chunky.

L'Humus de Peoples Pharmacy. *Peoples Pharmacy Hummus*

I know, if you live in Austin, you can buy it already made, but it's a lot more fun when you prepare your own, especially if you feel creative and want to add your own ingredients. This recipe is loaded with fiber as well as good olive oi and garlic.

Servings: 4

Prep Time: 20 min.

INGREDIENTS

- 1 can (15 oz) organic garbanzo beans, drained, but save the canning water
- 2 garlic cloves, chopped
- 6 Tbsp garbanzo canning water
- 3 Tbsp fresh lemon juice
- 3 Tbsp extra virgin olive oil
- ¾ tsp sea salt, fine
- ¼ tsp cayenne pepper

- 2 Tbsp tahini paste (sesame butter)
- Paprika powder
- 6 Pita breads

PROCEDURE

- Preheat your oven at 350°F to toast the pita bread.

- Drain the garbanzo beans, Saving the liquid. Place the garbanzo beans, garlic, garbanzo juice, lemon juice, olive oil, salt and pepper in the bowl of a food processor.

- Pulse to get the ingredients together, then switch to continuous speed and puree.

- Add the tahini and continue to process until smooth.

- Place in a beautiful colorful bowl; make a concentric swirl with a teaspoon and sprinkle with paprika powder.

- Cut the pita bread in 8 triangular pieces. Toast in your oven for about 8 minutes at 350F or until golden brown. Use to scoop the hummus.

✓ Chef's tip: You can vary this recipe by adding roasted red bell peppers, or black olives, or sun-dried tomatoes.

Fromage de Chèvre Fondu sur Pain aux Noix. *Melted Goat Cheese on Walnut Bread*

This wonderful appetizer is quick to prepare and sure beats your typical melted cheese sandwich. Try it with a mixed field green salad with walnuts. It makes a light but satisfying lunch all by itself.

Servings: 4

Prep Time: 10 min.

Cooking Time: 5 min.

INGREDIENTS

- **4 large slices of whole wheat walnut or olive bread (country-style bread is an acceptable substitute)**
- **4 small goat cheese buches (logs)**
- **Coarse black pepper**
- **Fresh savory herbs**

- **4 handfuls of mesclun (mixed field greens)**
- **1 Tbsp walnut oil**
- **½ fresh lemon juice**
- **Sea salt and freshly ground pepper to taste**

PROCEDURE

- Preheat your broiler. Set the oven shelf 3-4 inches from the broiler.

- Place your bread slices on a baking pan.
- Cut the goat cheese log in thick slices and place on the bread.
- Place pan in the oven and broil until the cheese melts slightly and starts coloring. Be careful not to burn the bread. Take out of the oven.

- In a separate bowl, place 4 handfuls of mixed field greens. Drop a few walnut pieces all over the salad. Drizzle with the walnut oil and lemon juice. Salt and pepper to taste. Toss lightly.

- Place each piece of bread with melted goat cheese at the center of each plate. Sprinkle with fresh savory herbs and surround with the tossed mixed field greens. Bite happily. Bon Appétit!

Petites Pissaladières aux Olives Niçoises. *Small Onion Tarts with Niçoises Black Olives*

This is the appetizer version of the classic pissaladiere Nicoise you can still find at the open farmer's markets all over Nice. They are typically criss-crossed with anchovies, but since I know most Americans' aversion to anchovies I did not put them in this recipe. Feel free to add anchovies if you are fond of them.

Servings: 4

Prep Time: 20 min.

Cooking Time: 10 min.

INGREDIENTS

- **2 Tbsp olive oil**
- **2 Tbsp butter**
- **2 large yellow or sweet onions, sliced thin**
- **2 garlic cloves, chopped fine**
- **½ tsp sea salt**
- **¼ tsp freshly ground black pepper**
- **2 tsp fresh thyme, chopped fine**

- **16 prebaked mini tart shells**
- **16 pitted olives Niçoises**

PROCEDURE

- Preheat your oven to 350°F.
- Heat a frying pan on medium heat. Add olive oil and butter and wait for it to sizzle.
- Add the sliced onions and chopped garlic. Sprinkle with sea salt. This will bring out the sweetness in the onions and help them to caramelize faster. Reduce heat.
- Add the black pepper and fresh thyme and keep cooking while stirring once in a while until the onions start turning light brown.
- Take off of the heat and allow them to cool down.
- If the mini tart shells are not baked, bake them according to the package instructions.
- When baked, fill each shell with a dollop of cooked onions and top with one pitted olive Niçoise per tart.

Soupes. Soups

Soupe aux Petits Pois et à la Menthe. *Green Pea Soup with Mint*

This soup is not made with split peas. It is made with tender sweet green peas with a touch of mint and it's loaded with fiber and chlorophyll. I love peas!

Servings: 4

Prep Time: 10 min.

Cooking Time: 10 min.

INGREDIENTS

- **2 Tbsp extra virgin olive oil**
- **1 small white onion, peeled and sliced in half moons**
- **1-12 oz bag of frozen green peas, defrosted**
- **2 carrots, peeled and diced**
- **1 quart vegetable broth**
- **Sea salt and pepper to taste**
- **¼ cup chopped mint**
- **2 Tbsp green onions, chopped**

PROCEDURE

- Defrost your peas in advance.
- In a saucepan, heat the oil at medium heat; sauté the onion until softened.
- Add the peas and carrots; cook for 2 more minutes to blend the flavors. Add the vegetable broth. Bring to a boil, reduce heat and simmer for 10 minutes.
- You can finish this soup two different ways:
- Place all of your soup in a blender (in portions if your blender is too small) and blend with the mint. Top with chopped green onions.
- Process half of the soup with the mint until pureed. Add back in to the chunky half for an interesting texture (This is the way I like it.) Top with chopped green onions.
- Please note: If you reheat this soup, do not boil it, as it will turn the mint bitter.

✓ Chef's tip: This soup is as delicious hot or cold. Enjoy it with garlic croutons.
✓ If you choose, you can replace ½ cup of broth with buttermilk at the final mixing stage. It will make the soup creamier and add a little tartness to it.

Soupe de Sante Verte d'Alain. *Alain's Healthy Green Soup*

When I feel "barbouillé" or "pas dans mon assiette", like when I feel a cold or flu coming on, I take a large bowl of this soup, go to bed, sweat it out and I usually feel a lot better the next day. Since I always have these ingredients at hand, this soup is very easy to put together in a few minutes.

Servings: 1

Yield: 2 soup bowls

Prep Time: 5 min.

INGREDIENTS

- **2 cups filtered or spring water**
- **4 cups of mixed field greens, or any greens you happen to have**
- **8 broccoli or cauliflower florets**
- **1 carrot, sliced**
- **2 garlic cloves**
- **1 tsp fresh ginger**
- **1 Tbsp fish oil**
- **1 Tbs miso paste**
- **1 tsp sea salt**
- **½ tsp cayenne pepper**
- **1tsp turmeric spice**

PROCEDURE

- Bring water to boil.

- Meanwhile, put all the ingredients listed in your blender's jar. Be creative and add any fresh vegetables you have in your fridge. What you put in is probably what you need.

- If you want it to be thicker, you can add 1 cup of cooked rice, a small cooked sweet potato, or even a raw egg for additional protein.

- Pour hot water over the ingredients and start blending slowly, then at high speed until finely pureed.

- Enjoy hot and go to bed to detox your body with a good sweating.

✓ Chef's tip: This is a hot but raw soup. The water is boiled but the vegetables are not cooked which makes it a raw soup. All the vitamins, minerals and chlorophyll are fully active and ready to help you feel better. Enjoy!

Soupe de Fanes de Carottes et Patate Douces. *Carrot, Carrot Greens, and Sweet Potato Soup*

This soup is loaded with vitamin B from the carrots and sweet potatoes. You also get a nice amount of chlorophyll from the carrot greens and leeks. I hope the color does not turn you off (greenish orange) because it is a very tasty and healthy soup.

Servings: 4

PROCEDURE

Prep Time: 15 min.

Cooking Time: 30 min.

INGREDIENTS

- **2 Tbsp extra virgin olive oil**
- **2 Tbsp butter**
- **2 or 3 white parts of leeks, sliced thin (about 2 cups)**
- **1 tsp sea salt**
- **The greens of a fresh organic bunch of carrots (6 to 8 carrots)**
- **4 medium sweet potatoes, cut into 1 inch cubes**
- **6 to 8 carrots, sliced**
- **1 ½ quart water or vegetable broth, cold**
- **2 tsp sea salt**
- **1 tsp ground black pepper**
- **2 Tbsp butter**

- In a large soup pot, heat the oil and butter.

- Sweat the leeks in the oil with the sea salt until they are tender.

- Add the carrot greens, and sauté for another minute.

- Add the sweet potatoes, carrots, water, salt and pepper.

- Bring to boil.

- Lower the heat and simmer for about 30 minutes or until the vegetables are tender.

- Process the soup in a blender one batch at a time.

- Pour into a soup tureen. Drop the additional butter and freshly chopped parsley for decoration

✓ Chef's tip: This recipe can be prepared with a pressure cooker. It will give the same results but faster. Finish the same way.

Soupe à l'Oignon au Vin Rouge. *Red Wine Onion Soup*

Traditionally, this soup was served as a mid-morning meal at bistros near Les Halles (the wholesale food market) in Paris. In some establishments, they left some of the meat used for the broth in the soup for additional flavor. This is my version with red onions and red wine. It's a good soup to build your blood and keep you warm in the winter.

Servings: 4

Prep Time: 15 min.

Cooking Time: 45 min.

INGREDIENTS

- **1 quart beef broth**
- **2 tsp sea salt**
- **2 laurel leaves**
- **2 sprigs fresh thyme**
- **6 black peppercorns**
- **2 Tbsp olive oil**
- **2 Tbsp butter**
- **2 lbs red onions, sliced 1/2-inch thick**
- **4 garlic cloves**
- **1 tsp sea salt**
- **½ cup dry red wine**
- **4 slices of baguette, sliced 1-inch thick**
- **2 garlic cloves**
- **2 cups grated Gruyère or Emmental cheese**

PROCEDURE

- Bring beef broth, sea salt, peppercorns and herbs to a boil.

- Remove from heat and let steep 10 minutes.

- Meanwhile, cook onions in oil and butter with the sea salt in a heavy medium pot over medium heat, stirring occasionally with a wooden spoon, until tender, about 15 minutes.

- Add wine to onions and boil until reduced to half its volume, about 1 minute.

- Strain broth through a sieve into onion mixture and simmer, covered, for about 30 minutes to allow all the flavors to blend. Adjust seasoning if needed.

- Preheat broiler.

- While the broiler is heating, toast 4 baguette slices in your toaster. Grate fresh garlic cloves over the toasted bread.

- Ladle hot soup into 4 ceramic bowls set on a sheet pan.

- Place toasted baguette slices on top of the soup and sprinkle each with 1/2 cup cheese.

- Broil about 4 inches from heat until the cheese gratinée turns golden brown, about 2 minutes.

- ✓ <u>Chef's tip</u>: The trick here is to cook the onions and garlic until they are slightly caramelized. That is what gives this soup its flavor. The salt added to the cooking onion help bring out their sweetness and accelerate the caramelization process. The red wine adds another layer of flavor.

- ✓ If you prefer a sweeter taste, feel free to substitute sweet Vidalia onions for red onions.

- ✓ Some chefs like to add the bread slices without toasting them. I not only prefer mine toasted; I like to scrub fresh garlic over it to add a hint of Provencal flavor. I also like the still crunchy mouth feel of the toasted bread while eating my soup. Enjoy!

Soupe de Lentilles à la Tomate et aux Épinards. *Lentil Tomato Soup with Spinach*

I love lentils. This is a vegetarian version of a traditional lentil soup. If you wish, you can add cubed ham to make it more of a meal.

Servings: 4

Prep Time: 15 min.

Cooking Time: 30 min.

INGREDIENTS

- **1 Tbsp extra virgin olive oil**
- **½ a medium white onion, chopped**
- **2 garlic cloves, minced**
- **1 celery stalk**
- **1 tsp sea salt**
- **1 tsp dried oregano**
- **1 tsp dried basil**
- **1 dried bay leaf**
- **½ tsp black pepper, ground**
- **1 cup dry green lentils**
- **2 large tomatoes or 1 can (15 oz) of crushed tomatoes**
- **2 carrots, diced**
- **1 quart organic vegetable broth**
- **½ cup baby spinach, sliced**

PROCEDURE

- In a large soup pot, heat oil over medium heat.

- Add onions, garlic, celery and salt; cook until all vegetables are tender.

- Stir in the bay leaf, oregano, and basil; cook for 2 minutes.

- Add in vegetable broth, lentils, carrots, and tomatoes. Bring to a boil.

- Reduce heat, and simmer for at least 30 minutes.

- When ready to serve, stir in sliced spinach and finish cooking until the spinach wilts but still is green, about a minute. Enjoy!

✓ Chef's tip: I personally like to keep this soup as is but if you wish, you can puree half of it to make it smoother.

Soupe Provençale a la Sauge et Ail. *Provencal Sage and Garlic Soup*

This old Provencal recipe has been considered a healing soup for generations. It is a good soup to have after too many libations, or when you're feeling a cold coming on. It is also thought to be anti-anemic and anti-spasmodic. It is supportive of heart health, stimulates bile secretions and has positive effects on gastric ulcers. It is a simple soup but has complex healing abilities.

Servings: 1 serving of two bowls

Prep Time: 15 min.

Cooking Time: 25 min.

INGREDIENTS

- **1 pint cold filtered water**
- **1 pinch coarse sea salt**
- **6 garlic cloves,**
- **4 slices country style bread**
- **4 Tbsp grated Gruyere cheese**
- **8 fresh sage leaves (or 2 tsp dried crushed sage)**
- **1 bay leaf**
- **Ground black pepper to taste**
- **2 Tbsp extra virgin olive oil**

PROCEDURE

- In a stainless steel pot, bring cold water to a boil with garlic cloves and sea salt. Once boiling, lower the heat and let it simmer, covered, for 15 minutes.

- Meanwhile, toast the bread slices with grated Gruyere. Let cool.

- When the soup has cooked for 15 minutes, add the sage and bay leaf. Let steep covered for about 10 minutes. Take the sage and bay leaves out. Adjust the seasoning with fine sea salt and freshly ground black pepper.

- When ready to serve, place 2 slices of the toasted bread at the bottom of the plate or bowl, add 1 tablespoon of olive oil, and ladle 1 cup of soup over it all. Enjoy your first soup bowl. Repeat the same process for the second serving. A Votre Santé!

Soupe Traditionnelle de Lentilles du Puy. *Traditional Du Puy Lentil Soup*

Green lentils from the town of Puy in the Auvergne region are so appreciated in France that we call them "poor man's caviar". They are small, round, and green, and are well known for their exceptional flavor and texture. They have been granted the same special status (AOC - Appellation d'Origine Contrôlée) by the French government as some wines. They can be found in America at specialty food markets.

Servings: 4

Prep Time: 10 min.

Cooking Time: 20 min.

INGREDIENTS

- **½ lb Puy lentils, or French green lentils**
- **1 quart cold water**
- **¼ lb of bacon, sliced 1/2 inch**
- **1 carrot, diced small**
- **1 large onion and 1 stalk of celery, diced small**
- **2 cloves of garlic, chopped**
- **2 cups chicken or vegetable stock**
- **Water to cover**
- **1 sachet of thyme, rosemary, bay leaf**
- **2 tsp sea salt**
- **½ tsp ground black**

PROCEDURE

- Spread your lentils on a large white plate or platter to check for possible small pebbles. Rinse in cold water.

- Bring lentils to a boil in a saucepan and immediately remove from the burner.

- Drain the lentils and run cold tap water over them until the water runs clear. Set aside

- Meanwhile, clean and dice your vegetables.

- In a soup pot, start cooking the bacon at medium heat to render the fat.

- Add the diced carrots, onion, celery, and garlic until the vegetables begin to release their moisture and start becoming tender.

- Add the lentils and stock. Add water to cover the lentils by 1 inch. Add bouquet garni (thyme, rosemary and bay leaf or their dried equivalent) Season as necessary with salt and pepper.

- Cook on medium heat until the lentils are tender, about 20 minutes. Taste for seasoning. Enjoy!

pepper

✓ <u>Chef's tip</u>: You may add butter and/or Dijon mustard to the finished lentils for a bit more dimension.

✓ If you are vegetarian, you may omit the bacon and replace the bacon fat with olive oil. Replace the chicken broth with vegetable broth.

Soupe au Pistou. *Pesto Soup*

This is a soup from my home town, Nice. The name "pistou" comes from an old "Nissarde" (the local language that the old folks still speak) word describing the marble mortar used to crush the basil paste that goes into the soup. That paste took on the name of the contraption used to make it. This soup is an entire meal. Eat it with toasted baguettes slices, rubbed with fresh garlic dropped in the soup.

Servings: 4 to 6

Prep Time: 20 min.

Cooking Time: 1 hour

INGREDIENTS

Soup ingredients:

- 2 quarts water
- 8 oz cured or smoked ham, cubed
- 1 cup dried Lima beans
- ½ cup dried red beans
- 4 medium potatoes, peeled and cubed
- 1 cup haricots verts, cut in fourths
- 2 ripe tomatoes, peeled and cubed
- 3 zucchini, cubed
- 1 eggplant, cubed
- 4 garlic cloves, peeled and crushed
- 2 Tbsp coarse sea salt

PROCEDURE

- Soak dried Lima and red beans overnight. Next morning, drain and rinse two times.

- In a large Le Creuset (enameled cast iron) soup pot, bring the water, ham and soaked beans to the boiling point.
- Lower the heat and cook covered for 20 minutes.

- Meanwhile, prepare your vegetables. The easiest way to peel your tomatoes is to blanch them in boiling water for a minute or until the skin separates from the fruit and drop in ice water. Allow to cool and peel. After the first 20 minutes, add all your prepared vegetables, crushed garlic and sea salt.
- Cook for another 20 minutes.

- Check your potatoes for doneness. When tender, you have two choices: you can leaves them as is, cubed. Or, using a skimmer, you can press the cooked potatoes through it to create a thicker soup. I personally like it that way. Another way to do it would be to puree your potatoes with some of the soup broth in a blender and pour it back into the

- ½ cup penne or shell pasta

Pistou Ingredients:

- 2 garlic cloves, peeled and crushed
- 1 packed cup of fresh basil leaves
- ¼ tsp coarse sea salt
- 1 pinch freshly ground black pepper
- 2 ripe tomatoes, peeled, seeded and cubed
- 4 Tbsp extra virgin olive oil

soup.
- Add the pasta and cook for another 10-12 minutes until the pasta is done.

How to prepare your pistou: there are 2 ways:

- The old-fashioned way: If you're lucky to own a marble mortar and pestle, this is the recommended way of doing it. At the bottom of the mortar, crush the garlic cloves with the pestle, add the sea salt and basil leaves and continue to crush. Add the tomatoes and black pepper. Continue to crush. Finally, add the olive oil in a light stream and finish to blend with the pestle. Add to finished soup. See Chef's tip below.
- The modern way: Using a blender, place the olive oil, garlic, basil leaves, sea salt, and pepper in the bowl and blend thoroughly. Add the tomatoes and finish blending. Add to finished soup. See Chef's tip below.

✓ Chef's tips: Very important: Add the pesto paste only at the end jus before serving and never boil the soup with the pesto in it. It will turn the soup bitter.
✓ Some chefs like to add grated parmesan cheese into their pesto. In Nice, we do not, as it tends to denature the pure basil flavor. If you want grated parmesan, add it on top of your soup just as you're ready to eat.
✓ Note: Some purists will scream bloody murder, but you have to remember that every chef will have his own interpretation of classics. Typically, Soupe de Pistou is made with lamb shank or ham on the bone. I have found that smoked or cured ham gives perfectly good results while cutting down the cooking time by at least 2 hours.

Soupe Minestrone Printanière. *Spring Vegetable Minestrone*

This Italian recipe is very much in favor in the South of France, to the point of making it our own with a few changes. Like the Soupe au Pistou, it is considered a whole meal, to be enjoyed with family and friends.

Servings: 6-8

Prep Time: 20 min.

Cooking Time: 35 min.

INGREDIENTS

- ¼ cup olive oil
- 2 small leeks, white and light green part only, washed and diced
- ½ small white onion, diced
- 4 garlic cloves, minced
- 2 medium carrots, diced
- 2 celery stalks, diced
- 2 quarts chicken or vegetable broth
- 1-15 oz canned Roma tomatoes, drained and chopped
- 1 parmesan rind (about 4 oz)
- 2 yellow squash, cut into half moons
- 2 small zucchini, cut into half moons
- 3 cups Swiss chard, cleaned, stemmed

PROCEDURE

- Heat the olive oil in a large pot over medium heat; add leeks, onion, garlic, carrots and celery; cook while stirring once in a while until your vegetables are soft.

- To that pot, add the broth, tomatoes and Parmesan rind. Bring to a boil, lower the heat and simmer for 15 minutes.

- Add the squash, zucchini and greens. Add salt and pepper. Cook another 15 minutes.

- Remove the pot from the heat. Take the parmesan rind out of the pot. Add the beans and stir. Adjust seasoning as you see fit.

- Serve in hot soup plates or bowls. Add a dollop of pesto on top.

and cut into ½-inch strips

- 1 Tbsp sea salt
- 1 tsp black pepper, freshly ground
- 1-15 oz can of cannellini beans, drained and rinsed

To finish Minestrone

Cilantro pesto for garnish

- 1 bunch cilantro, rinsed
- ¼ bunch parsley, rinsed
- ½ cup pine nuts
- 2 cloves garlic, minced
- ½ cup parmesan cheese, grated
- ¾ cup extra virgin olive oil

How to prepare the pesto:

- The old-fashioned way: Using a marble mortar and pestle, crush the garlic cloves with the pestle, add the sea salt, cilantro and parsley leaves and keep on crushing. Finally, add the olive oil in a light stream and finish blending with the pestle. Add to the finished soup when serving.

- The modern way: Place the oil, garlic, cilantro and parsley leaves, pine nuts and parmesan in your blender's bowl and blend thoroughly. Add to finished soup when serving.

Soupe de Fèves Fraiches. *Fresh Fava Bean Soup*

This is a simple but not quite traditional way to prepare a soup with fava beans at their peak of freshness. If some people from Provence read this recipe, they might cringe, as fava beans are typically eaten raw (like edamame beans) with a sprinkle of "fleur de sel"(sea salt) and a piece of fresh "pain de campagne".

Servings: 4

Prep Time: 15 min.

Cooking Time: 40 min.

INGREDIENTS

- **2 Tbsp extra virgin olive oil**
- **1 large sweet onion, diced small**
- **2 garlic cloves, minced**
- **1 quart vegetable broth**
- **1 large Yukon Gold potato, cubed**
- **1 lb fresh fava beans, shelled**
- **2 tsp sea salt**
- **1 tsp freshly ground black pepper**
- **2 Tbsp butter, cut into small pieces**
- **1 Tbsp green onions, minced**

PROCEDURE

- Heat the oil at medium high heat in a large soup pot. When the oil sizzles when water is sprinkled over it, add the chopped onions and garlic, and cook until tender.

- Add the vegetable broth and the cubed potato. Cook at a simmer for 20 minutes or until the potatoes are tender but not falling apart.

- Add the fresh-shelled fava beans to the soup and cook another 5 minutes with salt and pepper. Check if the beans are tender.

- Process in batches in the blender until pureed. Pour back into the pot. Bring back to a gentle simmer, add butter and minced green onions. Serve hot.

✓ Chef's tips: If you cannot find fresh fava beans, you can substitute ½ lb of dried fava beans. Soak them overnight a day ahead of time in filtered or spring water. Rinse them twice before using. Add the dried beans to the stock twenty minutes before adding the cubed potatoes. Do not cook the soaked beans with salt; it will prevent them from becoming tender. Season after the beans are fully cooked.

Soupe Gaspacho. *Gazpacho Soup*

As most of you probably know, this is a classic Spanish soup but is appreciated during the hot summer all over the Mediterranean basin. This is a simple recipe but the results will depend largely on the quality of your fresh vegetables.

Servings: 4

Prep Time: 20 min.

Cooking Time: 20 min.

INGREDIENTS

- **4 genuinely ripe medium tomatoes (local and in season is best)**
- **2 medium cucumbers, sliced**
- **2 celery stalks, sliced**
- **4 Tbsp extra virgin olive oil**
- **2 Tbsp parley, chopped**
- **2 Tbsp fresh basil, chopped**
- **2 large garlic cloves, chopped**
- **1 Tbsp sea salt**
- **1 tsp black pepper, freshly ground**
- **Tabasco to taste**
- **1 slice of dried whole wheat bread, cubed (optional)**

PROCEDURE

- If you wish, you can peel your tomatoes by plunging them in boiling water for a minute or until the skin detach from the fruit; pick up with a slotted spoon and drop in a container filled with iced water; let cool and peel. See Chef's note below.

- You can also decide to take the seeds out. In that case, quarter your tomatoes and squeeze the seeds out.

- Place the quartered tomatoes, sliced cucumber and celery in the blender and process fine.

- Add olive oil, parsley, basil, cloves, salt and pepper and Tabasco to taste and finish blending.

- One trick I learned from a friend is to add cubes of dried whole wheat bread and blend with the soup at the end to thicken this wonderful soup. Adjust seasoning to taste.

- For best flavor, serve this soup at room temperature and sprinkle with chopped parsley.

Soupe Vichyssoise a la Citrouille. *Butternut Squash Vichyssoise Soup*

Traditionally, a Vichyssoise soup is a cold soup made with leeks and potatoes. To give you more vitamin B, I created this version with Butternut squash.

Servings: 4

Prep Time: 10 min.

Cooking Time: 25 min.

INGREDIENTS

- **4 Tbsp butter**
- **1 white onion, peeled and chopped**
- **4 celery stalks, sliced**
- **4 leeks, white part only, sliced**
- **2 medium Butternut squash**
- **1 sprig of fresh thyme**
- **1 Tbsp sea slat**
- **1 tsp black pepper, ground**
- **1 quart chicken or vegetable broth**
- **Additional water to cover the veggies, if necessary**
- **4 Tbsp heavy cream**
- **1 tsp of Gomasio per soup bowl (optional)**
- **Or a few thin slices of fresh chives**

PROCEDURE

- Wash, peel and slice all the vegetables. Peel the butternut squash, cut in halves and take the seeds out.
- Chef's tip: If they are very tender, I keep the skin on and process it with my Vitamix. More vitamin B for the taking!
- In a large pot, melt the butter. Add the sliced onion and sauté while stirring for about 2 minutes.
- Add the celery and leeks and sweat for another 3 minutes.
- Add the cubed squash and thyme; cover with the broth and additional water if needed.
- Bring to boil and simmer for another 20 minutes, until the squash pieces are melting.
- Take the thyme sprig out, and puree the soup with the heavy cream.
- Cool down for at least 2 hours; serve with a generous sprinkle of Gomasio, or, if you cannot find it, a generous pinch of finely sliced fresh chives.
- ✓ Chef's tips: Gomasio, a well-known condiment in macrobiotic cooking, is made of toasted sesame seeds ground in a mortar with sea salt. A very tasty and aromatic condiment.

Soupe Froide de Betterave et Yogourt. *Cold Beet Soup with Yogurt*

This is a very refreshing "sweet and sour" soup. I like it better cold, but feel free to try it hot. It's delicious either way.

Servings: 6

Prep Time: 20 min.

Cooking Time: 20 min.

INGREDIENTS

- **2 Tbsp butter**
- **1 white onion, peeled and sliced**
- **2 shallots, minced**
- **4 medium beets, peeled**
- **¼ tsp of cumin**
- **2 tsp sea salt**
- **½ tsp cayenne pepper**
- **1 quart vegetable broth**
- **2 cups plain, unsweetened fresh yogurt**
- **Minced fresh dill for the final touch**

PROCEDURE

- Melt the butter in a medium soup pot; add the onions and shallots and sauté at medium heat for about 2 minutes, or until tender.

- Add the cubed beets and spices; add the vegetable broth and bring to boil; simmer for 30 minutes or until tender.

- There are two ways to finish this soup:

1. While still hot, process the soup with the yogurt. Refrigerate for at least 2 hours. Serve in white soup bowls. Sprinkle with fresh dill.

2. Process the soup without the yogurt. Cool down for at least 2 hours. Serve in white soup bowl. Spoon the yogurt over the soup and sprinkle with fresh dill.

✓ Chef's tip: Remember what I said in the ingredients section? Make sure to buy only unsweetened and unflavored natural or organic yogurt. That's the friendliest for your intestinal flora.

Soupe Froide d'Épinards et d'Avocat. *Cold Spinach and Avocado Soup*

Another one of my favorite cold soups. It is loaded with fiber, chlorophyll, healthy fats and it's very, very green. It tastes great and is very healthy for you. To dry the spinach, my grand-mother use to send me outside to shake the water out the "panier a salade". She used to just shake it hard but my favorite way of getting the water out was to turn round and round until my head was spinning. If I was lucky, I managed not to drop the salad in the process or else I would need to run real fast to avoid "une calotte" (a smack in the back of the head).

Servings: 4

Prep Time: 10 min.

INGREDIENTS

- 1 cup vegetable broth
- 2 Tbsp extra virgin olive oil
- 2 tsp lemon juice, fresh-squeezed
- 4 packed cups baby spinach, washed and dried
- 2 cloves garlic, chopped
- 1 tsp sea salt
- 1 large avocado, very ripe
- 2 Tbsp pine nuts, lightly roasted

PROCEDURE

- In your blender, combine the liquids: broth, olive oil and lemon juice; on top, press the spinach leaves, chopped garlic and sea salt; process, stopping once in a while to make sure to push the spinach leaves back into the mix.

- Peel and pit your avocado; add to the mix and finish blending. If necessary, adjust the thickness with a little more broth.

- Serve in white soup bowls and sprinkle pretty roasted pine nuts on top.

✓ Chef's tip: to toast the pine nuts, you can sauté them in a dry frying pan very carefully. Or better yet, roast them in your toaster oven at 350°F for about 8 minutes.

Accompagnements. *Side Dishes*

Recette Facile d'Alain de Riz et Haricots a la Tomate. *Alain's Easy Tomato, Rice and Beans Recipe*

This one-pot side dish is a simple recipe I put together when I need a side dish full of helpful fiber. You get it from the rice and the beans and, to make it tasty, I added the tomatoes and herbs. The kombu adds goodness from the sea.

Servings: 4

Prep Time: 10 min.

Cooking Time: 30 min.

INGREDIENTS

- **1 cup long-grain brown rice**
- **3 cups filtered water**
- **1 inch kombu seaweed (optional), soaked and cut in small pieces**
- **1-15 oz can Amy's Organics Vegetarian Chili**
- **1-15 oz can Muir Glen crushed tomatoes with basil**
- **2 Tbsp extra virgin olive oil**
- **1 Tbsp herbs de Provence mix**
- **1 tsp sea salt**
- **½ tsp cayenne pepper**

PROCEDURE

- If you choose to use the kombu – which I recommend – break off a one inch piece and soak for a few minutes to soften. Drain and cut in small pieces.

- Place your rice in a bowl full of water. Swirl around to wash it. Drain in a colander and run cold water over it to rinse it some more. Place in a 2-quart saucepan. Add 3 cups of filtered water. Add the kombu pieces and bring to a boil. Lower the heat to a gentle simmer and cook, covered, for about 20 minutes. Do not overcook. Keep your rice al dente. Let sit covered for another 10 minutes.

- While your rice is cooking, mix together the vegetarian chili mix, crushed tomatoes, olive oil, salt and pepper in a separate pot. Bing to boil, turn down the heat, and simmer for as long as the rice.

- When the rice has rested, mix the rice in to the tomato and beans mixture. Adjust seasoning and enjoy.

Flageolets Verts au Thym et Pignes de Pin. *Green Flageolets with Thyme and Pine Nuts*

Flageolets are green tender white beans shelled before full maturity. When I was a little kid, Mamie would ask me to help her take them out of their shells. Who's got the time now? You can find them flash frozen or canned. Try this recipe for a change; they will melt in your mouth.

Servings: 4

Prep Time: 20 min.

Cooking Time: 20 min.

INGREDIENTS

- **8 oz of thick-sliced bacon, cubed**
- **1 small onion, chopped**
- **2 garlic cloves, minced**
- **2-15 oz cans of flageolets, drained, or 1-12 oz bag frozen flageolets**
- **The juice of 1 lemon**
- **¼ tsp dried thyme**
- **Sea salt and pepper to taste**
- **Extra virgin olive oil**
- **4 tsp pine nuts**

PROCEDURE

- In a large pan, sauté the bacon cubes until melted. Set the bacon aside but save the fat.

- In the same pan, cook the onions and garlic until extremely soft.

- Add the drained or frozen flageolets, the lemon juice, thyme, salt and pepper and sauté gently for 10 minutes to allow the flavors to blend.

- When ready to serve, place on each warm plates, drizzle with olive oil and sprinkle with pine nuts. Enjoy!

✓ Chef's tip: This bean dish is traditionally served with roasted leg of lamb but also goes well with turkey.

Salade Chaude de Pois-Chiches d'Helene. *Helene's Hot Chickpea Salad*

Helene (my mother-in-law) used to make this simple but very healthy salad for us once in a while. Of course, she used to cook her own chickpeas, but to make your life easier, we're going to use canned chickpeas. Ah oui! The modern times require a shortcut once in a while as long as the quality does not suffer.

Servings: 4

Prep Time: 10 min.

Cooking Time: 10 min.

INGREDIENTS

- **2-15 oz canned organic chickpeas in their juice**
- **2 oz extra virgin olive oil**
- **2 Tbsp red wine vinegar**
- **1 small white onion, chopped fine**
- **3 garlic cloves, chopped fine**
- **1 Tbsp Herbes de Provence mix**
- **½ tsp sea salt**
- **¼ tsp cayenne pepper**

PROCEDURE

- Pour the chickpeas and their juice in a saucepan. Bring to boil, then turn off the heat. Set aside to keep warm.

- Meanwhile, prepare the salad dressing with the olive oil, vinegar, onion, garlic, herbs of Provence, salt and pepper.

- Drain the chickpeas and toss with vinaigrette while still warm.

✓ Chef's tip: Although not traditional, feel free to add sliced almonds or chopped walnuts to this dish to add more mono-unsaturated fat and fiber to this warm salad.

✓ I like to eat this salad by itself with grilled or canned sardines.

Artichauts à la Barigoule. *Artichoke Hearts a la Barigoule*

This dish can only be made with young and tender small artichokes in season. Helene whispered to me that her recipe was inspired by a famous local restaurant. She did not tell me which one. I will try to honor her spirit with this version rebuilt from memory.

Servings: 4

Prep Time: 20 min.

Cooking Time: 90 min.

INGREDIENTS

- **12 small young artichokes**
- **9-12 small white mushrooms, cleaned and chopped**
- **2 garlic cloves**
- **4 parsley sprigs**
- **3 slices of whole wheat bread**
- **2 Tbsp extra virgin olive oil**
- **¼ tsp dried thyme**
- **½ tsp sea salt**
- **Freshly ground black pepper to taste**
- **2 medium white onions, diced**
- **2 carrots, peeled and diced**
- **4 Tbsp extra virgin olive oil**
- **1 bay leaf**
- **1 cup filtered water**

PROCEDURE

- Trim the crust off the bread slices. Soak in water.
- Cut the artichokes' stems and save for later. With a small knife, trim the outer leaves and the stem. With a teaspoon, scoop out the center leaves and "hair". Place in water with vinegar to keep them from darkening.
- In a food processor fitted with the metal blade, place the sliced mushrooms, chopped garlic and parsley. Squeeze the water out of the bread and break off into the food processor. Pulse carefully. We want the ingredients to be chopped, not turned into a paste. Place these ingredients into a mixing bowl. Add the 2 Tbsp of olive oil, thyme, salt and pepper and blend well. Fill each artichoke with 2 teaspoons of "farce" (stuffing).
- Place the stuffed artichokes carefully in a Le Creuset or Dutch oven pot. Place the saved stems between the artichokes to stabilize them. Add the chopped onions, carrots, water and bay leaf. Drizzle the olive oil all over the artichokes. Cook for 1 ½ hour on the stove at medium-low until the artichokes are tender. Enjoy hot.

Topinambours a l'Ail a l'Étouffée. *Braised Garlic Roasted Jerusalem Artichokes*

This unjustly treated vegetable tastes like a cross between a potato and a celeriac. Since it does not contain any starch, it is a good vegetable for diabetics to cook with. Here's a simple but tasty recipe for you to try.

Servings: 4

Prep Time: 10 min.

Cooking Time: 20 min.

INGREDIENTS

- 1 ½ lbs Jerusalem artichokes
- 2 Tbsp extra virgin olive oil
- 4 cloves garlic, minced
- Sea salt and pepper to taste
- 2 Tbsp fresh parsley, chopped

PROCEDURE

– Peel the Jerusalem artichokes and slice across into equal rounds.

– Place in a pot with cold water. Bring to boil. Boil for 5 minutes. Drain.

– In a Le Creuset or Dutch oven pot, heat the oil at medium heat; add the garlic and cook until blond; add the drained artichokes. Sauté for another 5 minutes to meld the flavors. Lower the heat, cover and cook another 10 minutes until they are gold-colored and tender.

– When serving, sprinkle with chopped parley.

✓ Chef's tip: Use as an intriguing replacement for potatoes.

Patates Nouvelles Rôties aux Romarin. *Oven-roasted Rosemary New Potatoes*

I honestly don't remember where I learned this recipe, but I absolutely love it. It is a simple dish, full of the aromas of my Provence. The potatoes are melt-in-your-mouth tender, yet slightly crunchy from the sea salt.

Servings: 4

Prep Time: 10 min.

Cooking Time: 30 min.

INGREDIENTS

- **1 lb baby Yukon Gold potatoes or red potatoes**
- **2 Tbsp extra virgin olive oil**
- **2 Tbsp melted butter**
- **4 sprigs fresh rosemary, leaves separated from the branch**
- **2 tsp coarse sea salt**
- **1 tsp coarse black pepper**

PROCEDURE

- Preheat your oven at 400°F

- In a large bowl, mix together the olive oil, melted butter, fresh rosemary leaves, sea salt and black pepper.

- Cut your potatoes in halves or quarters depending on their size.

- Toss the potatoes in the flavored oil/butter mix.

- Place in one layer on a baking pan.

- Bake for 30-40 minutes (depending on potatoes size) or until the edges of the potatoes are turning golden brown.

✓ Chef's tip: Don't even think about using dried rosemary. There is no comparison in flavor. If you do, I will take you out of my will.
✓ This simple side dish is wonderful with lamb, roasted chicken or really any meat.

Portobello Farcis au Jambon. *Ham-stuffed Portobello Mushrooms*

I love the meaty flavor of Portobello mushrooms. Mushrooms are loaded with healing qualities but this dish is so good, you'll never know it's also good for you.

Servings: 4

Prep Time: 20 min.

Cooking Time: 40 min.

INGREDIENTS

- **8 medium Portobello mushroom heads, cleaned**
- **3 slices of whole wheat bread, trimmed**
- **½ cup milk**
- **2 Tbsp extra virgin olive oil**
- **2 shallots, minced**
- **2 slices of oven-roasted ham, chopped fine**
- **2 eggs**
- **½ tsp dried thyme or 1 tsp fresh thyme**
- **Sea salt and pepper to taste**
- **2 Tbsp butter**

PROCEDURE

- Preheat oven to 350°
- Trim the bread and soak it in the milk.
- Clean the mushrooms. Separate the stem from the "chapeau" (head).
- Dice the mushroom stems finely. Place in a mixing bowl. Squeeze the milk out of the bread and chop the bread finely. Add to the bowl. Beat the eggs; add to the bowl. Mix all these ingredients together with the thyme, salt and pepper.
- Peel and mince the shallots; chop the ham finely. In a frying pan on medium heat, sauté the shallots in olive oil; add the ham and cook until blond, about 5 minutes.
- Add bowl's mixture and cook another 10 minutes while stirring once in a while.
- Meanwhile, sauté the mushroom heads in butter, 2 minutes on each side until gold-colored. Repeat this operation if necessary.
- Place the sautéed mushroom heads in a roasting pan. Fill each mushroom head with about 2 tablespoons of stuffing. Bake for 20-25 minutes until the filling is golden brown.

✓ Chef's tip: Serve this dish with roast beef, bison meat or turkey.

Gnocchis Forestière. *Gnocchis with Mushroom Sauce*

Of course, you can make the gnocchis from scratch but trust me, unless you're an accomplished chef, it's a pain in the tablespoon. Buy them already made and enjoy the time saved in your kitchen. This side is wonderful with venison.

Servings: 4

Prep Time: 20 min.

Cooking Time: 20 min.

INGREDIENTS

- **2 lbs premade gnocchis**
- **8 oz small Crimini mushrooms**
- **4 oz dried cèpes or morilles mushrooms**
- **2 Tbsp extra virgin olive oil**
- **4 oz bacon, cut into pieces**
- **10 shallots, sliced**
- **3 small white onions, sliced in half moons**
- **1 cup dry white wine**
- **Sea salt and pepper**
- **10 parsley leaves, chopped**
- **2 bay leaves**
- **2 thyme sprigs**
- **3 Tbsp butter**
- **1 pint water**

PROCEDURE

- Soak the dried mushroom in warm water. After a while, rinse two times in cold water to make sure no sand is left. Drain and pat dry. Slice thin; set aside.
- Cut the bottoms off the crimini stems. Rinse in cold water and drain. Pat dry with paper towels. Cut in quarters.
- Peel and chop the onions and shallots. Chop the parsley. Cut the bacon.
- In a medium Le Creuset French Oven or Dutch oven, heat the oil over medium heat. Sauté the bacon, add the shallots and onions; cook a few more minutes until the onions are golden. Add the white wine and simmer until reduced in half.
- Meanwhile, in a frying pan on medium heat, melt the butter; add the quartered crimini, cook until the mushroom water is almost evaporated. Add the soaked mushrooms and cook for 2-3 minutes.
- Add the cooked mushrooms to the French oven; add the water, bay leaf and thyme. Cook covered for another 30 minutes at low heat.
- 15 minutes before the mushroom sauce is ready, cook the gnocchi according to the package's instructions. Drain the gnocchis and mix with the mushroom sauce.

Haricots Verts Rôtis aux Noisettes. *Roasted Haricots Verts with Hazelnuts*

Haricots verts are a thinner and more tender French version of green beans. This simple recipe is a nice way to discover them. I like the crunchy note added by the nuts. It is loaded with fiber, chlorophyll and mono-unsaturated oil from the hazelnuts.

Servings: 4

Prep Time: 10 min.

Cooking Time: 20 min.

INGREDIENTS

- **1 lb haricots verts**
- **3 Tbsp extra virgin olive oil**
- **1 tsp apple cider vinegar**
- **2 shallots, diced**
- **2 garlic cloves, chopped**

- **¼ cup hazelnut, toasted and chopped**
- **2 Tbsp fresh parsley, chopped**
- **½ tsp sea salt**
- **½ tsp freshly ground black pepper**

PROCEDURE

- Preheat your oven to 400°F.
- Toast the hazelnuts carefully until golden color, about 8 minutes.
- Typically, because haricots verts are so thin, they do not need to be trimmed, but you may have to trim a few of them. Cut them in half lengthwise.
- In a medium-sized bowl, whisk together the olive oil, apple cider vinegar, shallots, garlic, salt and pepper. Toss the haricots verts in this mix.
- Spread on a baking sheet and roast until tender but still crunchy, about 15-20 minutes.
- Take the beans out of the oven. While still warm, add the parsley and hazelnuts. Toss lightly and adjust seasoning.

✓ Chef's tip: This dish goes well with meatloaf, white fish or an egg dish.

Ratatouille. *Ratatouille*

This wonderful dish is the essence of Provence. The best time to prepare it is in the Summer when the tomatoes are full of flavor. If you want to prepare it at other times, I recommend using Muir Glen organic crushed tomatoes with basil. I know, it's a sacrilege, but it helps you savor this dish in all seasons. You can savor ratatatouille as a main dish, soup, side dish, or as a great pizza topping. Here's the version Helene taught me. Enjoy!

Servings: 4

Prep Time: 20 min.

Cooking Time: 1 hour

INGREDIENTS

- **½ cup vegetable broth**
- **3 Tbsp extra virgin olive oil**
- **1 medium white onion, peeled and cut in half moons**
- **2 garlic cloves, minced**
- **1 small green bell pepper, cut in thin slices**
- **1 small red bell pepper, cut in thin slices**
- **3 small eggplant, cut into 1 inch pieces**
- **3 medium zucchini, cut into 1 inch pieces**
- **3 large perfectly ripe tomatoes, or 1-28 oz Muir Glen Organics**

PROCEDURE

- Peel and chop onions and garlic. Toss together in a bowl and let sit for 5 min.

- Cut green and red bell peppers, take the seeds out, cut in four sections and slice thin.

- In a large skillet or pot, heat the vegetable broth and olive oil over medium-high heat; add the onions, garlic and bell peppers and sauté for 5 minutes, or until tender.

- Add the eggplant, zucchini and tomatoes (or canned tomatoes); mix well and cook for 10 more minutes until they start to soften.

- In a separate bowl, mix the tomato paste and red wine together. Stir in the parsley, basil, Provence herbs and spices.

- Add this flavorful mix to the vegetables and stir well. Lower the heat to simmer and continue to cook, covered, one more hour until all the vegetables are melted, like a stew or thick soup.

**crushed tomatoes
with basil**

- 3 oz tomato paste
  (skip if you use ripe
  fresh tomatoes)
- ½ cup red wine (the
  secret ingredient)
- 1 Tbsp fresh parsley,
  chopped fine
- 1 Tbsp fresh basil,
  chopped fine
- 1 Tbsp Herbes de
  Provence blend
- 1 tsp sea salt
- ½ tsp freshly ground
  black pepper

- Serve in white porcelain bowls to show off the ratatouille's bright colors (remember, we eat as much with our eyes as with our mouth) and sprinkle with a few fresh parsley leaves.

✓ Chef's tips: This dish can be a satisfying dish by itself, eaten warm or at room temperature. The flavors seem to bloom better at these temperatures than when hot.

✓ It also is a wonderful side dish with a sautéed filet of white fish.

✓ Another trick I learned from Helene is to prepare or buy a par-baked pizza crust and top it off with ratatouille mixed with one beaten egg and bake. The ratatouille tends to be runny so the egg holds it together. Sprinkle your favorite grated cheese on top: Romano, parmesan, or Swiss. Enjoy!

Viandes. *Meats*

Filets Mignons d'Agneau aux Épinards et Légumes Frais.

Filets Mignon of Lamb with Sautéed Spinach and Spring Vegetables

This is a very nice Spring recipe for lamb filets. Ask your butcher to cut the lamb filets for you. (You may have to special order in advance). This is where having a friendly butcher simplifies your life. Don't forget to tip him for Christmas!

Servings: 4

Prep Time: 20 min.

Cooking Time: 20 min.

INGREDIENTS

- **2 Tbsp olive oil**
- **2 Tbsp butter**
- **8 lamb filets**
- **2 thyme sprigs**
- **Sea salt**
- **Ground black pepper**
- **1 carrot, peeled and diced small**
- **1 turnip, peeled and diced small**
- **1 zucchini, unpeeled and diced small**
- **½ cup dry white wine**
- **2 Tbsp butter**
- **1 pound baby spinach**

PROCEDURE

- Using a Le Creuset cast iron enamel roaster with a lid (or a Dutch oven), melt the butter in the olive oil. Salt and pepper the lamb filets. Sauté them for 2 minutes on each side. Add the thyme, cover the pot and continue to cook for another 4-5 minutes.
- Take the meat and thyme out and reserve on a hot plate in a warm place. Deglaze the meat juices with the white wine. Add the small diced vegetables and cook another 5-6 minutes while stirring until tender.
- In a separate frying pan, sauté your spinach in melted butter until tender.
- When ready to serve, place the sautéed spinach on the lower portion of a hot plate; with a slotted spoon, top the cooked spinach nicely with the sautéed vegetables (drain and save the sauce). Place the lamb filets on the top portion of the plate and coat with the sauce and Voila!

Daube Provençale d'Agneau au Vin Blanc. *Provencal Lamb Stew with White Wine*

This recipe needs to marinate overnight. It will improve the meat flavor and tenderize the meat. To make sure the final result is fork tender, it needs to be cooked for a long time at low temperature.

Servings: 4-6

Prep Time: 30 min.

Cooking Time: 90 min.

INGREDIENTS

First day

- **1 lamb shoulder, deboned by your butcher**
- **6 oz shallots, peeled and chopped (about ¾ cups)**
- **4 garlic cloves, peeled and sliced**
- **4 carrots, peeled and cut in sticks**
- **4 small "pickling" onions**
- **1 celery stalk, chopped fine**
- **2 parsley sprigs with leaves**
- **1 tsp coarse sea salt**
- **½ tsp ground black pepper**
- **2 pinches grated or ground nutmeg**
- **6 juniper berries,**

PROCEDURE

- The day before preparation, ask your butcher to debone a nice lamb shoulder for you. If he's very nice, you can even ask him to cut the meat into 1-inch cubes.

- In a ceramic or enamel pot, put together the meat cubes, the chopped shallots, the sliced garlic cloves, the carrot sticks, the small white onions, the chopped celery, the parsley sprigs (whole with leaves), the coarse sea salt, the ground black pepper, the grated nutmeg, the crushed juniper berries, the thyme sprig, the bay leaves and the white wine.

- Stir well together; cover and set aside overnight at room temperature (if you feel more comfortable, you may refrigerate overnight but the marinade won't work as well and it will take longer to cook the next day).

- The next day, retrieve the meat, set aside on a plate; drain the marinade vegetables, herbs and spices in a colander set over a bowl. Set aside.

- In a French Le Creuset enameled pot or a

crushed

- 1 thyme sprig
- 2 bay leaves
- 1 bottle dry white wine (from Provence if possible)

Next day

- 2 Tbsp extra virgin olive oil
- 2 Tbsp butter
- 8 oz natural bacon, cut in small pieces (1/2 a lb)
- Additional vegetable or beef broth (as needed)

Dutch oven, heat the oil and butter at medium heat; sauté the bacon pieces until stiff; add the meat and color on all sides for about 10 minutes, stirring once in a while.

- Add the marinated vegetables; cook for another 10 minutes and finally add the wine to cover all the ingredients. If that is not enough liquid, you may add vegetable or beef broth to make sure to cover by one inch.

- Lower the heat; cover the pot and cook for at least 1 hour 30 minutes or until the meat is fork tender. Enjoy!

✓ Chef's tip: Serve with bow tie pasta or oven roasted rosemary new potatoes (see recipe)

✓ Unlike other recipes, there is no need to flour the meat to color it.

Daube de Bœuf à la Provençale. *Provencal-style Beef Stew*

My mother-in-law, Helene, prepared this dish wonderfully. Unfortunately, she passed away before I could ask her for her secrets. I suspect it had a lot to do with the well-seasoned special "daube" pot she used. After long research, this is the version I feel tastes the closest to her divine stew. This is a meal to share with friends around a lively table. It adds to the goodness of this dish.

Servings: 4

Prep Time: 40 min.

Cooking Time: 4-5 hours

INGREDIENTS

- **2 pounds of beef stew meat: shank or chuck, cut into 3 ounce pieces (ask your friendly butcher)**
- **2 Tbsp olive oil**
- **2 medium onions, peeled and sliced thin**
- **3 carrots, peeled and sliced thin**
- **1 celery stalk, sliced thin**
- **2 garlic cloves, peeled and sliced thin**
- **2 parsley sprigs with their leaves**
- **6 whole peppercorns, crushed coarsely**
- **2 pinches of coarse sea salt**

PROCEDURE

- In a large enameled cast iron pot, toss the meat along with the vegetables, herbs, spices, salt and pepper; sprinkle with the olive oil and cover with the red wine. Stir together well. Cover and marinate at least 6 hours, or overnight at room temperature. Note: If you feel uncomfortable with leaving this marinade out overnight, refrigerate overnight but the flavors will not develop the same way. If you are marinating during the day, stir every two hours.

- The next day, take the meat out and put aside; strain the marinade, saving the vegetables and the liquid separately. Dry the pot to be reused right away.

- In that same pot, melt the pork fat (or butter), and cook the cubed bacon and meat together for about 5 minutes; add the drained vegetables and cook for another 5 minutes; finally, cover with the marinade liquid. Bring to a gentle boil. If you own a heat disperser, place it on the flame and keep the heat to the level where the stew is barely simmering.

- 1 knife tip of ground nutmeg
- 4 juniper berries, crushed coarsely
- 1 fresh orange peel, cut in strips
- 2 cloves
- 2 fresh thyme sprigs
- 2 bay leaves
- 1 bottle of deep dark red wine with strong tannins

- 2 Tbsp organic pork fat or butter
- 2 oz lean bacon in one thick slice, cut into dices

- 4 cups of large egg noodles, macaroni or bow tie pasta, cooked in a large pot of salted water.

- Cook covered for 4 to 5 hours until the meat is falling apart.

- When the meat is ready, cook your noodles in a large pot of salted water for 12 minutes or al dente. Drain. Place the cooked pasta on the bottom of your serving dish, and cover with the stew. Serve pasta and meat separately and allow each guest to help themselves to their heart's content.

✓ Chef's tip: One of the old folks' secrets when it comes to this stew is that you should top the stew pot with a large plate and fill it with a cup of red wine (or water). When the wine or water evaporates, add some more until the meat is cooked. What this does is to allow the steam from the stew to condense against the cool lid filled with liquid and fall back into the stew to develop a better flavor. I believe in this method, too. As a matter of fact, if you visit the South of France, you can buy a "daube" earthenware pot with a special lid that allows you to add liquid on top.

✓ Chef's tip: Some chefs believe that adding tomatoes or tomato paste to this "daube" makes it more special. As you already know, every chef will add his own twist to any recipe. I don't recall Helene using tomatoes in hers, but if it works for you, give it a try and let me know how it tastes.

Pain de Viande aux Herbes du Midi. *Southern France Meat Loaf*

This is my version of a meat loaf with "herbes de Provence". It adds a special flavor "du Midi" to a classic recipe. I usually serve this with new potatoes oven-roasted with rosemary.

Servings: 1 loaf. 8 people

Prep Time: 20 min.

Cooking Time: 55 min.

INGREDIENTS

- **2 lbs grass fed ground beef**
- **8 strips organic or nitrite-free bacon**
- **2 Tbsp extra virgin olive oil**
- **1 medium white onion, chopped fine**
- **2 garlic cloves, chopped fine**
- **8 oz Crimini mushrooms**
- **2 large eggs**
- **1 slice whole wheat bread, processed into crumbs**
- **2 tsp sea salt**
- **2 tsp chives, sliced**
- **1 tsp dried sage**
- **1 tsp fresh thyme, chopped fine**
- **1 tsp black pepper**

PROCEDURE

- Preheat your oven to 350°F.
- Cut the bacon in pieces and fry until crispy; drain and set aside.
- Peel and chop the onion and garlic. Finely chop the mushrooms. Heat the olive oil, sauté the onion and garlic until softened; add the mushrooms and cook well. Reserve.
- In a large stainless steel bowl, combine the ground beef, bread crumbs, eggs, bacon, and cooked mushrooms with their juice, and all the herbs and spices. Mix well.
- Spray your meat loaf pan with olive oil spray. Add the meat mix; press down. Place in the oven on a baking sheet.
- Bake for about 45 minutes or until internal temperature reaches 160°F (use a meat thermometer). Take the meat loaf of out the oven. Let it sit for 10 minutes before slicing and serving.

✓ Chef's tip: Top each slice with your favorite heated tomato sauce and serve with oven-roasted rosemary new potatoes.

Roti de Bison Sauce Chasseur. *Bison Roast with Hunter's Sauce*

This is a wonderful twist on a classic Fall recipe. Usually, it is prepared with deer meat. Try this version with mashed potatoes. It's so good, you will lick your chops.

Servings: 4

Prep Time: 20 min.

Cooking Time: 20 min.

INGREDIENTS

- 1 ½ pound bison roast (ask your friendly butcher to tie it up for you)
- 1 tsp sea salt
- ½ tsp freshly ground black pepper
- 2 Tbsp olive oil
- 2 Tbsp butter
- 3 large tomatoes
- 2 Tbsp olive oil
- 1 tsp chopped parsley
- ½ garlic clove, chopped
- ½ lb white button mushrooms
- 1 Tbsp butter
- 1 Tbsp olive oil
- 2 tsp chopped shallots
- ¼ cup Cognac
- ¼ cup dry white wine

PROCEDURE

- Preheat your oven to 400°F.
- Salt and pepper your bison roast.
- Heat the olive oil and butter a 5-6 quart Le Creuset or Dutch oven pot; brown the roast on all sides.
- Place in the oven and cook covered for 30 minutes.
- Meanwhile, drop your tomatoes in a large pot of boiling water. Cook about 1 minute until the skin separates. Drop in ice water and peel.
- Cut tomatoes into small dice. Sauté in olive oil with the chopped parsley, garlic, salt and pepper. Crush your tomatoes with a fork as you cook them. Process in your blender and strain to make a "coulis" (sauce).
- Clean your mushrooms; slice thin and sauté in a little olive oil and butter with the shallots. Add a little salt and pepper. Deglaze them with the cognac and white wine. Bring to boil and cook to reduce the liquid by half.
- Add your tomato "coulis"; bring back to a simmer and let your sauce ingredients blend with each other for a couple of minutes. Adjust seasoning if necessary.
- Slice your roast; serve two slices per person on a hot place. Coat with the sauce

Ragout de Bison aux Canneberges. *Bison Cranberry Stew*

Since we can now find cranberries in France, I decided to experiment with it and came up with this recipe. If you don't feel like eating turkey at Thanksgiving, enjoy this recipe with your family.

Servings: 4

Prep Time: 20 min.

Cooking Time: 2 hours

INGREDIENTS

- 1 Tbsp extra virgin olive oil
- 1 Tbsp butter
- 1 medium size onion, chopped
- 2 cloves garlic, sliced thin
- 1 lb bison stew meat, cut in one inch cubes by your friendly butcher
- 1 cup dry red wine

- 3 cups organic beef broth
- 2 tsp sea salt
- ½ tsp freshly ground black pepper
- 2 Tbsp organic Worcestershire sauce
- 1 ½ tsp paprika
- 2 whole cloves
- 2 bay leaves

PROCEDURE

- Put olive oil and butter in a 5 or 6 quart enameled cast iron pot (Le Creuset) or a Dutch oven.

- Over medium heat, brown the bison cubes. Remove the meat and set aside. In the same fat, sauté the onion and garlic until soft. Deglaze with the red wine. Add the meat back into the pot; stir the meat to coat with the wine.

- Add the beef broth, salt, pepper, paprika, Worcestershire sauce, cloves and bay leaves. Bring to a boil and reduce the heat; cover and simmer for 1 hour, stirring every 20 minutes or so.

- Add carrots, potatoes, cranberries and celery. Bring to a boil, reduce heat, cover and cook for another 30 to 45 minutes, or until potatoes are fork tender. Add beef broth if necessary.

- Adjust seasonings — more salt, pepper, and Worcestershire sauce may be required.

- Using a separate bowl, prepare a thickener by gradually stirring the cold water into the cornstarch.

- Increase heat so that the stew maintains a moderate boil. Stir the stew continuously while blending in half of the thickener. After two minutes, add more thickener and continue to cook and stir until desired consistency is reached.

- **4 carrots, peeled and sliced thin**
- **4 medium Yukon Gold potatoes, cut into large cubes**
- **1 cup cranberries (fresh or frozen)**

- **¼ cup corn starch**
- **1 cup cold water**

- Remove bay leaves and serve.
- This stew reheats well.

✓ <u>Chef's tip</u>: You can serve this wonderful stew with wide egg noodles.
✓ <u>Chef's tip</u>: You can prepare this stew the day before. Refrigerate. Skim the fat off the top and re-heat gently.

Cotes de Porc Grillées à la Moutarde et Sauge. *Grilled Pork Chops in Mustard and Sage*

This very aromatic recipe is very easy to prepare. This is the French way of flavoring your pork chops. I use a Le Creuset cast iron grilling pan; this way I avoid the bad side effects of grilling over charcoal.

Servings: 4

Prep Time: 10 min.

Cooking Time: 10 min.

INGREDIENTS

- **4 pork chops**
- **4 tsp Dijon mustard**
- **Sea salt to taste**
- **Freshly ground black pepper to taste**
- **Fresh sage leaves, chopped**
- **Macadamia or grape seed oil**

PROCEDURE

- The day before, using a brush, spread mustard on both sides of your pork chops.

- Salt and pepper them to your taste; sprinkle fresh chopped sage leaves all over the chops, pressing them in lightly.

- Place your chops on a plate; drizzle them all over with macadamia or grape seed oil. Wrap them in plastic film and store them in your refrigerator overnight.

- The next day, take your pork chops out of the refrigerator at least one hour before cooking to allow them to come back up to room temperature.

- Preheat your cast-iron grilling pan at medium temperature on the stovetop and cook your chops the way you like them best.

✓ Chef's tip: I also like my chops sprinkled with fresh rosemary, a very aromatic and healing herb.

Cotes de Porc aux Pommes à la Cannelle. *Baked Pork Chops with Apples and Cinnamon*

In France, cooking pork with apples is a wonderful way to add sweetness to an otherwise bland meat. It is a tasty and warming Autumn dish.

Servings: 4

Prep Time: 20 min.

Cooking Time: 30 min.

INGREDIENTS

- **4 medium pork chops**
- **2 Tbsp butter**
- **½ cup dry white wine**
- **Sea salt to taste**
- **Freshly ground black pepper to taste**
- **4 celery leaves**
- **4 bay leaves**
- **2 Granny Smith apples, cored and diced**
- **2 celery stalks, chopped fine**
- **1 Tbsp butter, cut in small pieces**
- **1 Tbsp brown sugar**
- **4 oz grated Swiss cheese**

PROCEDURE

- Preheat your oven to 400°F.

- Butter an ovenproof enameled cast iron or glass pan.

- Place your pork chops in the pan, leaving a little space in between; Sprinkle with salt and pepper to taste. Top each chop with a celery leaf and a bay leaf.

- In a separate bowl, toss together the diced apples, the chopped celery, butter, and brown sugar. Add this mix to the pan with the pork chops, placing some of the mix between the pork chops.

- Bake together for about 30 minutes (depending on the size of your chops). Check for doneness.

- Take the pan out of the oven. Set your oven on broiler. Take out the celery and bay leaves. Sprinkle the Swiss cheese over your pork chops. Put back in the oven and broil until the cheese is melted and turns golden brown.

✓ Chef's tip: This recipe is also very tasty with veal chops.

Cotes de Veau aux Pignons de La Côte d'Azur. *Veal Chops with Côte d'Azur Pine Nuts*

This way of preparing veal chops adds a touch of sweetness. The nuts add a welcome crunchiness and the mushroom an earthy touch.

Servings: 4

PROCEDURE

Prep Time: 15 min.

Cooking Time: 15 min.

INGREDIENTS

- 4 – 8oz veal chops
- Sea salt to taste
- 2 Tbsp extra virgin olive oil
- 2 Tbsp butter
- 4 Tbsp Banyuls wine (sweet wine) or port wine
- 1 cup organic beef broth
- 1 pound Crimini mushrooms, sliced thin
- 4 oz pine nuts
- 1/2 cup heavy cream
- Freshly ground black pepper to taste
- A few parsley leaves, chopped fine

- Lightly salt the raw veal chops.
- Clean and slice the mushrooms. Chop the parsley.
- Heat the oil and butter in a large frying pan.
- Cook at medium heat for 3-4 minutes on each side.
- When the meat is golden, take the chops out of the pan; discard the fat, but keep the scrapings on the bottom of the pan.
- Put the chops back into the frying pan and deglaze with the Banyuls wine (or port wine); add the beef broth; increase the heat to reduce the sauce quickly.
- Add the sliced mushrooms, pine nuts and heavy cream. Let simmer a few minutes to allow the flavors to blend.
- Place the cooked chops on a hot serving platter; coat with the sauce; sprinkle with the chopped parsley.

✓ Chef's tip: These chops will go well with pan-fried sliced Yukon gold potatoes.

Filet de Chevreuil Sauce Grand Veneur. *Venison Filet with Grand Veneur Sauce*

This is a hunting season favorite in France. Save recipe for a special occasion, as it is rich and takes quite a while to prepare. Enjoy during the cool days of Fall.

Servings: 4-6

Prep Time: 30 min.

Cooking Time: 80 min.

INGREDIENTS

- 2 Tbsp olive oil
- 2 Tbsp butter
- 1 filet of venison, about 3 lbs (ask for the cuttings and bones for the sauce)

For the marinade

- 1 cup onions, peeled and chopped fine
- 1 cup carrots, peeled and chopped fine
- 1 celery stalk, chopped fine
- 2 shallots, sliced
- 1 garlic clove, peeled and crushed
- 1 bay leaf
- 1 thyme sprig
- 1 rosemary sprig
- 2 tsp sea salt
- 1 tsp coarse black pepper

PROCEDURE

- The day before, place the venison filet at the bottom of a large enameled cast iron Le Creuset French oven. Add the chopped onions, carrots, celery, sliced shallots, crushed garlic, herbs and spices.

- Then, add the olive oil, cognac, and red wine. Make sure the filet is covered with liquid; otherwise, turn over every hour. Marinade at least 6 hours or overnight at room temperature.

- The next day, take the meat out of the marinade and drain. Dry carefully. Strain the marinade over a bowl. Take out the herbs, set aside and save the liquid and other ingredients.

- In that same pot (cleaned and dried), heat the olive oil and butter. Cook the meat cuttings and bone(s) with salt and pepper. When colored, lower the heat to medium, add the herbs from the marinade and flour and continue to cook for another 5 minutes while stirring.

- Add the red wine vinegar and the drained wine from the marinade; Bring to boil and cook covered at low heat for 30 minutes.

- 2 Tbsp olive oil
- ¼ cup Cognac
- 1 bottle rich red wine such as Bourgogne

For the sauce

- 2 Tbsp olive oil
- 2 Tbsp butter
- Meat cuttings and bones
- 2 tsp sea salt
- ½ tsp ground black pepper
- ½ cup unbleached flour
- ½ cup red wine vinegar
- Red wine from marinade
- ¾ cup crème fraiche or heavy cream
- 4 oz bilberries or cranberries

Skim the floating scum off the top once in a while.

- Strain the sauce; add the cream and berries, cook another 5 minutes to allow the berries to pop.

- Heat your oven at 400°F.

- While the oven heats, take the deer meat and cook in the olive oil/butter until well colored on all sides.

- Place the deer meat in an oven-proof braising pan and cook for about 20 minutes (for rare, or longer if you wish). Once in a while, spoon the fat over the meat to keep it moist. Once cooked, wrap in a sheet of aluminum foil and let rest for 5 minutes inside the oven, heat turned off.

- When ready to serve, slice the deer meat, place on hot plates on top of cooked egg noodles. Cover with the meat and the noodles with the sauce. Enjoy!

Chevreuil aux Cerises et à l'Orange. *Venison in Cherry and Orange Sauce*

Another tasty Autumn recipe.

Servings: 4

Prep Time: 20 min.

Cooking Time: 60 min.

INGREDIENTS

- **1.5 lbs saddle of venison (ask your friendly butcher)**
- **4 juniper berries**
- **½ tsp dried thyme, ground**
- **Sea salt**
- **Ground black pepper**

- **2 Tbsp olive oil**
- **2 Tbsp butter**

- **4 oz untreated bacon, sliced thin (about 5 slices)**
- **1 oz of Better than Bouillon Beef stock and 2 cups of water, or, 2 cups organic beef broth**

- **1 can small cherries in light syrup, drained (save the**

PROCEDURE

- Preheat your oven to 450°F.

- Spike the meat with the juniper berries; rub with the thyme powder. Let the meat rest for 10-15 minutes. Take out the juniper berries. Salt and pepper the meat.

- Heat an enameled cast iron roasting pan (Le Creuset) on the stove; cook the meat in the oil/butter until well-colored. Carefully wrap the bacon over the cooked meat. Add the beef broth to the pan.

- Place the pan in the oven and cook for about 35 minutes. Every 10 minutes, open the oven and spoon the beef broth over the meat to keep it moist.

- After 30 minutes, take the bacon away from the meat. At that time, check how well the meat is done. It should be soft to the touch and still pink inside. When the meat is cooked to your liking, let it rest for 15 minutes in the oven, heat shut off and the door ajar.

- In a saucepan, mix the cherry juice into the corn starch while whisking. Add the grated orange peel. Bring to a boil gently, making sure the sauce is thickening.

juice)

- **2 tsp corn starch**
- **1 grated organic orange peel**
- **½ cup kirsch liquor (cherry brandy)**

- **8 oz egg noodles, cooked al dente**

- Add the cherries to the sauce; add the kirsch and mix in with the strained drippings from the oven pan.

- Place cooked egg noodles on the hot plates, top with 4 slices of the meat and coat with the sauce. Enjoy!

Volailles. *Poultry*

Salade de Poulet aux Raisins et Noix Rôties. *Chicken Salad with Grapes and Toasted Walnuts*

This is a recipe I created for People's Pharmacy. Our customers really enjoy it and come back for more every day at lunch.

Servings: 4

Prep Time: 20 min.

Cooking Time: 20 min.

INGREDIENTS

- 1 lb skinless chicken breasts, poached
- 1 stalk celery, chopped fine
- 1/3 cup grated carrot
- 1 Tbsp Dijon mustard
- ½ tsp sea salt
- ¼ tsp freshly ground black pepper
- 1 cup Spectrum organic mayonnaise (or your favorite brand)
- 4 oz seedless black grapes, washed and cut in half (about ¾ cup)
- 1 cup toasted walnut pieces

PROCEDURE

- **Poaching the Chicken:** The day before you plan to serve this salad, fill up a medium pot half way with hot water. Bring to boil on high.
- Place the chicken breast gently in the boiling water (do not burn yourself!). Keeping the heat on high, bring back to boil. Take pot off the heat. Check to make sure chicken is cooked but not overdone.
- Drain cooked chicken breasts into colander. Let cool to room temperature. Cut into ½ inch cubes. Let cool overnight or at least 2 hours.
- **Toasting the Walnuts:** Preheat your oven to 350°F. Spread walnuts pieces on a baking sheet. Place in oven. Roast for 5 minutes, turn the baking sheet around; roast another 5 minutes. Check for a light brown color and a nutty fragrance. Let cool before adding to salad.
- The next day put together the celery, carrot, Dijon mustard, salt and pepper, grapes, walnut pieces and mayonnaise in a large mixing bowl. Toss together gently. Add the chicken pieces and mix well. Enjoy!

Poulet Roti au Citron et aux Herbes Aromatiques. *Lemon and Herb Roasted Chicken*

The aroma of this simple dish as it cooks will charm your senses. On your plate you will enjoy the lemon-rosemary flavor combination. It goes well with oven-roasted rosemary new potatoes.

Servings: 4

Prep Time: 20 min.

Cooking Time: 20 min.

INGREDIENTS

- 1 medium (3.5-4 lbs) organic or free range chicken
- 2 lemon rinds, grated
- 4 garlic cloves, minced
- 2 tsp thyme, chopped fine
- 2 tsp rosemary, chopped fine
- 2 tsp sage, chopped fine
- 2 tsp sea salt
- 1 tsp black pepper, ground

PROCEDURE

- Preheat your oven at 400°F.
- In a small bowl, combine lemon, garlic, herbs and spices to form a slightly moist paste.
- Wash the chicken and dry thoroughly inside and out.
- Loosen the skin across the breast and then down around the legs and thighs using a chopstick, or with your fingers.
- Work the seasoning mixture under the skin and into the meat of the breast, legs and thighs and all over the outside skin as well.
- Season the cavity of the chicken with salt and pepper. Using butcher's string, truss the chicken tightly.
- Place the chicken in a roasting pan.
- Cook for 50-60 minutes, or until the internal temperature reaches 180°F on a meat thermometer inserted in the thigh. Remove from oven. Let rest for 10 minutes before cutting.
- Remove chicken and cut to a quarter chicken per person.

✓ <u>Chef's tip</u>: If you have only 2 people for dinner, ask your friendly butcher for one whole chicken breast with skin on and proceed the same way. Just reduce the cooking time to 35-40 minutes.

Dinde Rôtie aux Pruneaux et Pommes. *Roasted Turkey with Prunes and Apples*

I like this way of preparing turkey because of the sweet stuffing; it's like eating dinner and dessert at the same time. In France, we serve this meal with chesnuts and flageolets.

Servings: 8-10

Prep Time: 30 min.

Cooking Time: 4 hours

INGREDIENTS

- **1 turkey of about 8 lbs, with giblets**
- **½ stick softened butter**
- **3 Tbsp olive oil**
- **1 large onion, chopped fine**
- **2 garlic cloves, chopped fine**
- **1 cup finely chopped celery**
- **10 pitted prunes, chopped fine**
- **2 Granny Smith apples, cut in small cubes**
- **2 Tbsp chopped walnuts pieces**
- **2 slices whole wheat bread soaked in milk**
- **2 tsp dried thyme**
- **Sea salt and freshly ground pepper to**

PROCEDURE

– Preheat your oven at 300°F.
– Soak bread in milk. When soft, squeeze the milk out and crumble the bread.

Preparing the stuffing:

– Heat the oil in a sauté pan; add the onion and garlic and cook until soft; add the giblets, celery, prunes, cubed apples and walnuts; add the crumbled bread, thyme, salt and pepper. Continue to cook, stirring occasionally, until all the ingredients are softened.

Prepare the turkey:

– Salt and pepper the turkey inside and out.

– Fill the turkey cavity with the cooked stuffing. Truss tightly with butcher's string. With a brush, coat the turkey all over with softened butter. Place the turkey in a large Le Creuset French Oven or covered turkey roaster. Cover and cook at 300°F for one hour. Keeping the oven on, take the pot out of the oven and brush the turkey with its own juice using a pastry brush. (If you prefer, you may use a baster.) Add butter if needed. Place back in the oven and cook for another 3

taste

hours. Every 30 minutes or so, baste the turkey to keep it moist. 30 minutes before the end of cooking, increase the oven's heat to 350°F, take the cover off and finish cooking until the skin has a nice caramel color. To check for doneness, stick a small knife in the thick of the breast. If the juice comes out clear, your turkey is done.

- Remove the turkey from the oven. Let rest for 10-15 minutes. Slice and serve with the stuffing and the strained cooking juices.

✓ <u>Chef's tip</u>: If you wish to cook your turkey a day ahead, prepare as above and cook for 3 hours. Refrigerate overnight. The next day, heat your oven to 300°F and cook for another hour. Finish with another 30 minutes at 350°F.

Poissons et Fruits de Mer. *Fish and Seafood*

Ma façon rapide de préparer un filet de saumon. *Alain's Quick Way to Prepare Salmon Filet*

When I come back home from working all day in a professional kitchen and I want to eat my ration of fresh fish, this is the way I cook it. It is very tasty and very quick. Serve it with a composed salad and Voila! Dinner is served.

Servings: 2

Prep Time: 5 min.

Cooking Time: 3-4 min.

INGREDIENTS

- **2 beautiful salmon filets**
- **4 oz of your favorite salad dressing as a marinade or**
- **2 tsp extra virgin olive oil with your favorite herbs or spice blend**
- **Sea salt and freshly ground black pepper**
- **Your favorite mixed green salad with your favorite salad dressing**

PROCEDURE

- Preheat your (toaster) oven to broil for 5 minutes. Place a Le Creuset enameled cast iron pan, cast iron pan or heavy stainless steel frying pan in your oven and allow to heat for at least 10 minutes.

- Meanwhile, you can prepare your salmon (or any fish, really) one of two ways:

1. Brush the filets with your favorite vinaigrette on both sides. Place in a plastic bag and let marinade for 10 minutes.

2. Brush your filets with olive oil. Press them into your favorite herbs blend. Let sit for 10 minutes.

- When your pan is well heated, take it out of the oven with oven mittens and place your fish filets on the hot pan. Put back in the oven right away. Using a timer, cook for 3 minutes, or more depending on your filets' thickness. It's ready!

✓ Chef's tip: Actually, if you don't mind the bones, I prefer to get a slice of the salmon tail and cook it this way. It's more fatty, thus more moist… and it actually costs less.

Moules Provençales. *Provencal-style Mussels*

If you're fond of shellfish, this is a wonderfully aromatic recipe. You may need some expertise in opening the mussels, as they will refuse to cooperate.

Servings: 4

Prep Time: 60 min.

Cooking Time: 2-3 min.

INGREDIENTS

- **4 pounds fresh mussels, cleaned and picked by your friendly fishmonger**
- **½ a stick of butter at room temperature**
- **3 garlic cloves, chopped fine**
- **1 Tbsp chopped fresh parley**
- **1 tsp chopped fresh dill**
- **1 tsp sea salt**
- **½ tsp cayenne pepper**

PROCEDURE

- Ask your favorite fishmonger to clean your mussels. Make sure they are not opened, which means they are dead and not edible.
- Let your butter soften at room temperature. Chop the garlic, parsley, and dill finely and blend with the butter, then blend in the salt and cayenne. Set aside.
- Preheat your broiler. Move the oven shelf to about 3-4 inches from the broiler.
- With an oyster knife, open each mussel. Throw away half of the shell; keep the other half with the meat in it. Place on a baking pan or oven dish.
- When they are all opened, top the meat in the shell with the softened flavored butter with a small spatula or butter spreader.
- Broil for 2 minutes until gratiné. Be careful not to overcook or they will become chewy.

✓ Chef's tip: You may sprinkle the cooked mussels with additional chopped parsley for additional color.

Loup de Mer au Four au Blanc de Provence. *Sea Bass in White Provencal Wine*

This is a wonderful recipe for when you have guests. My mother used to make it only on very special occasions. Traditionally, this fish is served with quartered boiled or steamed potatoes tossed with garlic-parsley butter. Serve with the same wine you used for cooking the fish.

Servings: 4

Prep Time: 40 min.

Cooking Time: 75 min.

INGREDIENTS

- **1 whole 3-4 pound sea bass, scaled and cleaned**
- **2 Tbsp olive oil**
- **2 tomatoes, sliced**
- **4 stalks of fennel, sliced thin**
- **4 garlic cloves, minced**
- **4 shallots, minced**
- **1 lemon, sliced**
- **4 parsley sprigs**
- **2 bay leaves**
- **2 tsp sea salt**
- **8 black peppercorns**
- **1 cup dry white wine from Provence or other white wine**
- **1 cup water**
- **8 medium- sized potatoes, peeled and cubed**

PROCEDURE

- Preheat your oven at 400°F.
- Brush your oval Le Creuset roasting pan or oven dish with olive oil.
- In a large mixing bowl, place the sliced tomatoes, sliced fennel, chopped garlic, shallots, sliced lemon, parsley, bay leaf, salt and black peppercorns; add the dry white wine, water and the remaining olive oil. Toss all of these ingredients together.
- Place half of these ingredients at the bottom of your roasting pan.
- Lay the fish on top.
- Add the remaining ingredients to the fish. Pour the leftover liquid into the pan.
- Surround with the potatoes, peeled and cut in large cubes. Salt and pepper.
- Place in the oven and cook for 1 hour 15 minutes (or longer depending on the size of your fish). To keep the potatoes moist, baste every 20 minutes with the cooking juices.
- When ready, transfer the fish to a hot serving platter. Surround with the potatoes. Keep warm.
- Meanwhile, strain the remaining ingredients and reserve the cooking juices. Coat the fish and potatoes with this sauce.

Daurade Filets aux Herbes en Papillotes. *Sea Bream with Herbs cooked in Papillotes*

This is a very elegant and simple way to cook a fish while trapping all the flavors. To surprise your guests, ask them to pop open the top of the "papillotte" with their knife and inhale the wonderful "fumet" (smell). A lovely surprise!

Servings: 4

Prep Time: 10 min.

Cooking Time: 15 min.

INGREDIENTS

- **4 nice filets of sea bream, keep the skin on for additional flavor (you can substitute halibut or flounder)**
- **2 Tsp extra virgin olive oil**
- **8 thin lemon slices**
- **8 sprigs fresh thyme**
- **8 sprigs of parsley**
- **4 pinches of rosemary leaves**
- **Sea salt and freshly ground black pepper**
- **½ dry white wine**

PROCEDURE

- Ask your friendly fishmonger to scale and clean 2 sea breams and cut them into filets but ask for the skin to be left on.
- Preheat your oven at 400°F.
- Cut 4 large pieces of parchment paper 4 inches wider than your filets.
- Brush each sheet with olive oil. Place the filets at the center. Place 2 lemon slices, 2 thyme and parsley sprigs, a sprinkle of rosemary leaves, salt and pepper. Drizzle the white wine carefully over the fish.
- Now for the tricky part: Fold the paper over in a triangular shape. Then fold each side twice to seal the fish and ingredients inside the pouch. Cheating trick: the paper may be difficult for you to fold. Use a stapler if you need to. Just make sure to tell everyone to watch out for stray staples.
- Bake for 15-20 minutes and Voila!
- Serve with your favorite pasta tossed in butter and chopped parsley.

✓ Chef's tip: Some chefs prefer to use aluminum foil to form their papillotes. I am careful not to have my food in direct contact with aluminum as there are suspicions that cooking in or with aluminum could increase the chances of Alzheimer disease. Be safe and use baking paper.

Thon Façon Côte d'Azur. *Tuna Côte d'Azur-style*

Tuna is a very meaty fish, the closest to red meat. It needs strong flavors to work with. This recipe provides you all the scents of Provence.

Servings: 4

Prep Time: 20 min.

Cooking Time: 30 min.

INGREDIENTS

- **1-2 pounds tuna filet, about 1 ½ inches thick, cut into 4 filets by your friendly fishmonger**
- **1 Tbsp olive oil**
- **A few sprigs of savory**
- **A few sprigs of thyme**
- **A few rosemary leaves**
- **Sea salt and freshly ground pepper to taste**

Sauce:

- **3 Tbsp olive oil**
- **1 medium onion, sliced thin**
- **4 garlic cloves, minced**
- **1-28 oz can of Glen Muir crushed tomatoes with basil**

PROCEDURE

- Ask your friendly fishmonger to cut you an nice thick slice of tuna steak, cut into 4 filets.

Prepare the fish:

- Brush the tuna steaks with olive oil, then sprinkle the herbs all over them on both sides. Press them in. Let sit at room temperature for 3 to 4 hours.

Prepare the sauce:

- Heat the oil in a saucepan on medium heat, sauté the onion and garlic until soft but not caramelized. Add the canned tomatoes with the juice. Add the herbs, salt and pepper. Simmer for a while until the liquid has mostly evaporated.
- Lower the heat, add the chopped capers and black olives. Stir in gently. Adjust seasoning if necessary. Set aside.

Cook the tuna:

- Remove the herbs from the tuna. Sprinkle with salt and pepper.
- In a large frying pan on high heat, warm up the oil. Add your tuna filets and cook no more than 4 minutes per side. Remove the skin and serve.

- ½ tsp sea salt
- ½ tsp dried savory
- ½ tsp dried rosemary leaves
- ½ tsp dried thyme
- ½ tsp sea salt
- ½ tsp freshly ground black pepper
- 2 Tbsp capers, drained and chopped
- ½ cup black small olives Niçoises, drained and chopped fine

- 2 Tbsp olive oil
- Sea salt and freshly ground pepper to taste
- Chopped parsley

Serve the tuna:

- Place on heated plates, spoon the sauce over each filet and sprinkle with chopped parsley.

✓ <u>Chef's tip</u>: I serve this fish with oven-roasted Rosemary new potatoes. Délicieux!

Filets de Truites Amandine. *Trout Filets Amandine*

I love almonds. I love them in my desserts or cakes and I love them with my fish. This is a simple but tasty way to eat your almonds.

Servings: 4

Prep Time: 10 min.

Cooking Time: 10 min.

INGREDIENTS

- **2 rainbow trout, scaled and cleaned, cut in 4 filets. Ask your friendly fishmonger to keep the skin on**
- **½ cup sliced almonds**
- **2 Tbsp olive oil**
- **2 Tbsp butter**
- **Sea salt, fine**
- **Freshly ground black pepper**
- **1 lemon juice**
- **½ cup chopped parsley**

PROCEDURE

- In your toaster oven, toast the almonds until light brown. Set aside.

- In a frying pan on medium heat, heat the oil and butter until it sizzle.

- Add the filets skin side up. Cook for about 3 minutes. Flip over carefully. Cook for another 4 minutes or until done to your satisfaction.

- Transfer to a heated serving platter and keep warm.

- Meanwhile, deglaze the pan with the lemon juice and whisk to blend with the cooking juices.

- Pour over the filets. Sprinkle the toasted almonds and chopped parsley over the fish. Enjoy!

✓ Chef's tip: Traditionally, this dish is cooked with the butter heated the "beurre noisette" level, when it just starts to brown. If that's too tricky for you, just cook like above.

✓ Serve with lightly steamed haricots verts dressed with lemon vinaigrette.

Salades. *Salads*

Salade de Mesclun aux Pamplemousses avec Croutons. *Mixed Field Greens Salad with Grapefruit and Croutons*

The mesclun salad mix was invented by the monks of the Cimiez monastory in Nice. One of them decided to grow an assortment of local salad seeds in their "potager" (kitchen garden), then harvest them while still young and serve them with a drizzle of olive oil. It became customary to offer a basket of mesclun to their benefactors as a thank you gift. I like this salad for its lightness and freshness. It does not use vinegar but citrus fruit juice for the acidity in the vinaigrette. It is loaded with vitamin C and chlorophyll.

Servings: 4

Prep Time: 15 min.

INGREDIENTS

- **1 pound of mixed field greens or one premixed bag**
- **2 grapefruits, peeled and quartered**
- **½ of a rustic baguette bread, sliced**
- **2 garlic cloves, peeled**
- **½ cup freshly squeezed grapefruit juice**
- **½ cup freshly squeezed lime juice**
- **1 cup extra virgin olive oil**
- **½ tsp sea salt**
- **¼ tsp black pepper**

PROCEDURE

Croutons

- Slice the baguette bread into thin slices. Toast them lightly and rub with a garlic clove cut in half. Continue toasting to your taste.

Vinaigrette

- Squeeze and strain the grapefruit and lime juice into a small mixing bowl. Add the salt and freshly ground black pepper. Stream in the olive oil while whisking the vinaigrette.

To finish the salad

- Place the salad in a salad bowl.
- Peel and quarter the grapefruit on top of the greens.
- Drizzle the vinaigrette over it. Toss gently. Decorate with the garlic croutons.

Salade Niçoise. *Niçoise Salad*

Here's another classic from my hometown, Nice. Also called "la salade du soleil" (salad of the sun) in our region. It is loaded with fresh produce brought from the daily neighborhood open market or picked fresh from the garden. This salad will evolve with the seasons. It will be slightly different in Spring than in Summer. I will give you a modern version. Have fun and be proud of your own version. Needless to say, this is a whole meal enjoyed with family and friends.

Servings: 4

Prep Time: 40 min.

INGREDIENTS

- **1 head of fresh lettuce or your favorite garden salad**
- **8 heirloom tomatoes, firm and not too ripe**
- **½ lb of new small potatoes or small red potatoes**
- **4 oz haricots verts or green beans (about ¾ cup)**
- **2 small artichokes, peeled and sliced or 1 can artichoke hearts (optional)**
- **1 colorful pepper (green, red, yellow)**
- **8 oz canned tuna pieces in water**
- **1 celery branch with leaves**
- **2 green onions or 2 shallots**

PROCEDURE

- Cut the salad leaves from the core, wash and drain properly.
- Wash the tomatoes; cut them in 8 parts, do not slice them (it looks prettier and you won't have tomato seeds all over the salad). Sprinkle them with sea salt and let sit in your refrigerator.
- Hard-boil the eggs; cool and peel them and cut them in quarters.
- Cook the potatoes until tender but not too soft. Drain, cool and set aside. Cut in halves.
- Steam your haricots verts for 5 minutes or until al dente. Drain, cool, set aside. Cut in 2 inch pieces.
- Peel and mince the green onions or shallots.
- Place the anchovy fillets between two paper towels to pat them dry.
- Wash the pepper; cut the top off; take the seeds out and slice thin.
- Wash the celery and cut into small dice.
- If you wish to use fresh artichokes, pull the outer leaves out and with a small knife, cut out the outer part to expose the heart. Rub with a half fresh lemon all over to keep it from darkening. Slice thin and

To decorate your salad

- **6 eggs, hard-boiled**
- **2 oz small black olives Niçoises (about 1/3 cup)**
- **8 anchovies filets in olive oil, patted dry**

Red Wine Vinaigrette

- **8 Tbsp extra virgin olive oil**
- **2 Tbsp red wine vinegar**
- **½ tsp sea salt**
- **¼ tsp freshly ground black pepper**

reserve. Or drain canned artichoke hearts.

- Using a large deep platter or salad bowl, place the salad leaves at the bottom; add a layer of tomatoes, a few potato halves, a few cut haricots verts, a few slices of artichoke (optional), a couple of slices of colorful pepper, tuna pieces, a couple of pinches of diced celery and green onion slices.
- Repeat this operation until you run out of ingredients.
- Prepare your vinaigrette. Toss the composed salad gently.
- Decorate the top of your salad with hard-boiled egg quarters, small black olives and anchovy fillets.
- Bon Appétit!

✓ Chef's tip: If you want to prepare a luxury version of this salad, you can replace the canned tuna with fresh grilled tuna.

✓ Other options are fresh shelled green peas or beans, add a few leaves of parsley or basil; add finely minced garlic. You can use any salad greens you like or even mixed field greens (my favorite). Have fun and be creative. Just don't go too far out there or you will not be able to call it "Salade Niçoise" any more.

Salade Camarguaise. *Salad from the Camargue Region*

This salad was created using rice from the Camargue region of France. It is located west of Marseille where the Rhone and the Mediterranean sea meet. It's marshes are France's rice growing region. If you decide to visit, you will see the famous wild white horses and black bulls as well as the only French cowboys you'll ever see. Another example of a salad as a complete meal.

Servings: 4

Prep Time: 20 min.

Cooking Time: 15 min.

INGREDIENTS

- **1 cup long grain brown rice**
- **1 quart of water**

- **8 oz roast beef or chicken leftovers**

- **4 medium tomatoes, ripe but firm**
- **4 eggs, hard-boiled**
- **1 lettuce heart, washed and dried**
- **Fresh tarragon leaves**

- **2 Tbsp red wine vinegar**
- **1 tsp Dijon mustard**
- **Sea salt, pepper**
- **4 cornichons (tiny French pickles)**
- **8 Tbsp extra virgin olive oil**

PROCEDURE

- Rinse the rice in running water. In a medium pot, bring the water to boil. Add your rice and reduce the heat to low. Cook gently for about 15 minutes until "al dente". Rinse in cold water. Drain.
- Meanwhile, hard boil the eggs. Cool down and peel. Cut one egg in eight sections, chop the rest.
- Wash your tomatoes; cut into 8 sections.
- Wash and drain the lettuce. Cut the leaves and pat them dry. Thinly slice the leaves.
- Wash and dry the tarragon leaves.
- Chop the cornichons finely (small French gherkins pickled in vinegar).
- Cut your leftover meat in one-inch cubes.
- Prepare your vinaigrette by mixing first the mustard, cornichons, salt and pepper. Mix well. Add the vinegar and whisk together. Add streaming olive oil and mix well.
- To finish the salad, place half of the cooked rice at the bottom of a salad bowl; add the tomatoes, meat, chopped eggs, the other half of the rice and minced lettuce. Drizzle with vinaigrette and toss gently. Decorate with egg sections and tarragon leaves.

Salade de Radicchio, Orange Sanguine, Roquette et Olives.
Radicchio, Blood Orange, Arugula and Olive Salad

I love the subtle blend of bitter greens with the sweetness of the oranges and the saltiness of the olives. The sherry vinegar add a sweet and sour note to the flavor symphony.

Servings: 4

Prep Time: 20 min.

INGREDIENTS

- **3 Blood or Valencia oranges**
- **2 heads of radicchio salad (about 4 cups)**
- **1 bunch fresh arugula**
- **½ red onion, peeled and sliced thin**
- **½ cup pitted black olives Niçoise**
- **4 oz fresh goat cheese**

Vinaigrette

- **2 Tbsp sherry vinegar**
- **Sea salt and ground black pepper to taste**
- **¼ cup extra virgin olive oil**

PROCEDURE

Prepare the oranges

- Cut off both ends of each orange. On a cutting board, stand your orange on one end and peel the skin and white pith with a small paring knife cutting from top to bottom.
- Over a small bowl to catch the juice, cut each orange segment between the membranes to remove the segments. Let drop into the bowl. Squeeze the remains of the orange into the same bowl. Drain the segments and reserve the juice.
- Wash and drain your salad greens.

Orange-sherry vinaigrette

- In another small ceramic, glass, or stainless steel bowl, whisk together the sherry vinegar, 2 Tbsp of the reserved orange juice, salt and pepper and finally the olive oil.
- To serve the salad, place your radicchio and arugula salad leaves artistically on each plate. Top with the orange segments, sliced red onion and black olives. Drizzle with the orange-sherry vinaigrette and finish with slices of goat cheese.

Salade d'Asperges avec les Herbes du Jardin et Parmesan.

Asparagus, Garden Herbs and Parmesan Salad

The secret in this salad is to steam the asparagus very lightly until al dente. The fresh garden herbs will add that extra green kick and the parmesan its saltiness.

Servings: 4

Prep Time: 15 min.

Cooking Time: 4 min.

INGREDIENTS

- **1 bunch small asparagus spears**
- **½ cup flat leaf parsley, leaves only**
- **¼ cup fresh dill, leaves only**
- **¼ cup fresh mint, leaves only**

- **1 lemon zest**
- **1 lemon juice**
- **Sea salt and freshly ground pepper to taste**
- **4 Tbsp extra virgin olive oil**

- **¼ cup parmesan, shaved**

PROCEDURE

- In a large pot fitted with a steam basket, bring water to a boil.

- Meanwhile, take one asparagus tip; fold it until it breaks off the hard bottom naturally. Using this as a guide, cut the other spears with a chef's knife.

- When the water is boiling, place the asparagus tips in the steaming basket, cover and cook for 4 minutes only. Rinse in cold water, drain and pat dry.

- At the bottom of a salad bowl, whisk together the lemon juice, zest, salt and pepper and olive oil.

- Add the steamed asparagus tips and the herbs. Toss gently with the dressing. Decorate with the parmesan shavings.

Salade de Roquette, Melon de Cavaillon et Jambon Fume.
Arugula, Cavaillon Melon and Serrano Ham Salad

When prepared with a melon de Cavaillon, a small and sweetly tasty melon, this recipe brings me back home to Provence. Unfortunately, they are very difficult to find in America. Feel free to substitute with a small and very ripe Cantaloupe.

Servings: 4

Prep Time: 15 min.

INGREDIENTS

- **2 bunches arugula**
- **1 small ripe Cavaillon or Cantaloupe melon**

Vinaigrette

- **2 Tbsp fresh lime juice**
- **¼ tsp sea salt**
- **¼ tsp smoked paprika**
- **1 pinches cayenne pepper**
- **4 Tbsp extra virgin olive oil**

- **4 oz Serrano or other dry or smoked ham, sliced very thin**

PROCEDURE

- Wash the arugula; drain and pat dry.

- Cut the melon in half; scoop out the seeds. Cut in eight sections, peel the skin off and cube the meat.

- In a salad bowl, whisk all the vinaigrette ingredients together.

- Add the arugula and the cubed melon and toss gently.

- Place on serving plates. Top with two thin slices of Serrano or your favorite dry or smoked ham. Enjoy!

Salade de Mesclun avec Poires Concorde, Noix et Roquefort.

Mixed Field Greens with Concord Pear, Walnuts and Roquefort

I enjoy this fall salad for the added sweetness and crispiness of the pear, the slight bitterness and crunchiness of the walnuts and the creamy Roquefort. The raw, unfiltered apple cider vinegar is loaded with beneficial compounds such as potassium, minerals and live enzymes beneficial to the gut. A healthy gut makes a healthy body!

Servings: 4

Prep Time: 20 min.

INGREDIENTS

- **1 pound mixed field greens**
- **2 Concord pears**
- **½ cup walnut pieces**
- **½ cup Roquefort**

Apple Cider Vinaigrette

- **2 Tbsp raw, unfiltered apple cider vinegar**
- **¼ tsp sea salt**
- **2 pinches freshly ground black pepper**
- **4 Tbsp walnut oil**

PROCEDURE

– If needed, wash, drain and pat dry the salad.

– Wash your pears; quarter and core them; cut in half-inch slices. <u>Note</u>: I like to keep the skin on for extra fiber. You may peel them if you prefer.

– Whisk together your vinaigrette ingredients at the bottom of a salad bowl. Add the salad leaves, sliced pears and walnut pieces. Toss together gently.

– Place on plates and top with crumbled Roquefort. Enjoy!

✓ <u>Chef's tips</u>: Feel free to substitute the walnut oil with virgin macadamia oil or extra virgin olive oil.
✓ I love Roquefort for its sweetness, but any quality blue cheese is fine.
✓ You may toast the walnuts but be aware; it will bring out more of their bitterness.

Céleri Rémoulade et sa Sauce Yaourt. *Grated Celeriac Salad with Yogurt Dressing*

This is a classic French salad that makes good use of the unknown celery root. Traditionally, it is made with mayonnaise. I offer you a lighter and fresher version prepared with plain, natural yogurt. The natural tartness of yogurt compliments the celeri root perfectly. Celery root is a natural diuretic and yogurt is loaded with friendly bacteria.

Servings: 4

Prep Time: 20 min.

INGREDIENTS

- **1 large or 2 small, celery roots, washed and peeled**

Yogurt dressing

- **1 tsp Dijon mustard**
- **1 shallot, peeled and minced**
- **½ tsp sea salt**
- **2 pinches freshly ground black pepper**
- **1 cup plain, natural yogurt (not sweetened or flavored)**
- **Parsley leaves**

PROCEDURE

- Wash and peel your celery root(s). Cut into pieces small enough to fit your food processor feeding tube. Grate your celery using your food processor grating plate.

- In a medium bowl, whisk together all of the yogurt dressing's ingredients.

- Add the grated celery root and toss together.

- Decorate with a few parley leaves.

✓ Chef's tip: This salad is a perfect accompaniment to a fillet of broiled fish like tuna or salmon.

Salade de Lentilles du Puy aux Lardons et Jambon du Puy.
Lentil Salad with Bacon and Dried Ham

This salad is made with the famous Lentilles du Puy, also called the poor people's caviar . They are so special that the French government gave them the AOC (Appellation Controlee d'Origine) certification. These small green pulses stays firm when cooked and are loaded with fiber and minerals.

Servings: 4

Prep Time: 20 min.

Cooking Time: 20 min.

INGREDIENTS

- 1 cup Lentilles du Puy or other lentils
- 1 bay leaf
- 3 springs fresh thyme
- 2 oz natural bacon, cut in small pieces (3-4 slices)
- 1 onion, peeled and chopped fine
- 2 oz dried or smoked ham, cubed (1/3 cup)
- A few chervil leaves
- 1 Tbsp balsamic vinegar
- ¼ tsp Dijon mustard
- 1 small shallot, peeled and minced
- 3 Tbsp extra virgin olive oil
- Sea salt and black pepper to taste

PROCEDURE

- Make sure the lentils are clean of possible pebbles. Place them in a medium saucepan; add three cups of cold water. Bring to a boil and lower the heat. Cook for 20 minutes or until tender, but not mushy. Drain in a colander. Set aside in salad bowl.

- Meanwhile, in a frying pan, sauté the cut bacon until crispy. Take the bacon out and pat dry. Using the fat from the bacon, sauté the chopped onions. Place on top of the lentils. Add the cubed dried or smoked ham. Add the sautéed bacon.

- In a small stainless steel bowl, mix all of the vinaigrette's ingredients. Pour over the lentils, veggies, bacon and ham.

- Toss together gently. Decorate with a few chervil leaves.

✓ Chef's tip: If you do not live in a big city with fancy grocery stores, feel free to substitute with any good quality organic lentils.

Salade de Carottes, Ananas et Raisins Secs. *Carrot, Pineapple and Raisin Salad*

This is a sweet and tart salad. You can find it in all French "traiteurs" (caterers) windows but I added pineapple chunks to this recipe to make it more fun.

Servings: 4

Prep Time: 20 min.

INGREDIENTS

- ½ cup raisins
- 1 pound carrots, washed, peeled and grated
- 8 oz fresh pineapple chunks

Vinaigrette

- 1 oz fresh lemon juice
- 1 tsp sea salt
- ½ tsp cayenne pepper
- 2 Tbsp extra virgin olive oil

PROCEDURE

- Place your raisins in a small pan. Cover with water. Bring to boil. Take off the flame. Let soak while the rest of the salad is prepared.

- Wash, peel and grate your carrots with your food processor's grating plate.

- Cut both ends of your pineapple. Place it on a cutting board and cut the skin off from top to bottom with a sharp chef's knife. Cut into eight pieces; remove and discard the core. Slice pineapple into half-inch chunks. To make things easier, you may want to buy your pineapple chunks already pre-cut.

- Prepare the dressing at the bottom of your salad bowl. Whisk all the ingredients thoroughly.

- Add the carrots, pineapple chunks and drained raisins. Toss gently and enjoy!

✓ Chef's tip: If you feel adventurous and want to make this recipe more exotic, you may soak the raisins in rum. Just don't tell the kids.

Salade d'Épinards Jeunes aux Framboises et Amandes. *Baby Spinach Salad with Fresh Raspberries and Almonds*

This easy recipe is loaded with fiber, iron and vitamin K from the spinach, and powerful antioxidants from the raspberries. And such a beautiful plate to look at!

Servings: 4

PROCEDURE

Prep Time: 15 min.

- The baby spinach should come already washed. If not, wash, drain and pat dry.

INGREDIENTS

- 8 cups or one bag baby spinach
- 1 pint (8 oz) fresh raspberries
- 4 oz fresh goat cheese, sliced
- ½ cup slices almonds

- In a large salad bowl, whisk all your vinaigrette ingredients together.

- Add the baby spinach leaves, the fresh raspberries and the sliced almonds. Toss gently with the vinaigrette.

Raspberry vinaigrette

- Serve on beautiful white plates. Top with the goat cheese slices.

- 2 Tbsp raspberry vinegar
- 1 tsp Dijon mustard
- ¼ tsp Sea salt
- 1/8 tsp cayenne pepper
- 6 Tbsp extra virgin olive oil

- Bon Appétit!

✓ Chef's tip: Feel free to replace the sliced almonds with walnut or pecan pieces, or pine nuts.

Vinaigrettes and Sauces. *Dressings and Sauces*

Vinaigrette de Santé d'Alain. *Alain's Healthy Salad Dressing*

This is not a magic potion - like the one of Asterix and Obelix comic book fame (the fans will know what I'm talking about) - but pretty darn close. It is loaded with only ingredients known to help keep your heart healthy. Nothing but heart-healthy ingredients!

Servings: ~30

Prep Time: 15 min.

INGREDIENTS

- **1 cup apple cider vinegar or fresh lemon or lime juice**
- **4 cloves of fresh garlic, peeled and sliced**
- **1-2" piece of Ginger, peeled and sliced**
- **3 Tbsp Dijon-style Mustard**
- **1 tsp Sea Salt**
- **½ tsp Cayenne Pepper**

- **1 cup extra-virgin olive oil**
- **1 cup of flax seed oil for an extra boost of omega 3 fatty acids**

- **2 Tbsp Bragg's Liquid Aminos**

PROCEDURE

- Place the first set of ingredients in the blender. Blend at high speed until garlic and ginger are well processed.
- Meanwhile, measure olive oil and flax seed in the same measuring cup.
- Through the hole in the blender's lid, pour the oil slowly into the above mix until it's fully absorbed.
- If you want an additional burst of amino acids and additional flavor, add the Bragg's liquid aminos.
- Note: If you find this dressing a little too acid (I love it that way) you can change the acid to oil proportions from 1:2 to 1:3. That is 1 cup of acid (vinegar or lemon juice) to 3 cups of oil blend (for example, 2 cups Olive oil and 1 cup Flax Seed oil).

✓ Chef's tip: I prepare this size recipe and store it in the refrigerator in a squeeze bottle. That way, when I want to put together a quick salad, I just place some salad on a plate, shake the bottle of dressing and squeeze some of it on top of your salad. Voila!

Sauce Aïoli ou Ailloli. *Aïoli or Ailloli Sauce*

This is a classic cold Provençal sauce that is the favorite accompaniment to cold roast beef, steamed potatoes, or a piece of white fish. **Caution:** *this recipe is very garlicky. You can kiss the fish but not your better half unless you both ate the same sauce. To ensure it sets properly, make sure to have all the ingredients set at room temperature for at least one hour before preparing it.*

Servings: 8

Prep Time: 20 min.

INGREDIENTS

- **8 garlic cloves, peeled and minced**
- **½ tsp fine sea salt**
- **4 egg yolks**
- **¼ tsp freshly ground white pepper**
- **3 cups extra virgin olive oil**

PROCEDURE

- Peel the garlic and remove the germ.
- In a marble mortar, using a pestle, crush the garlic with the sea salt.
- Add the yolks, one by one, while turning in the same direction (pick one direction and stick with it through the whole process) for about 2 minutes. Let rest for 5 minutes (if you do not, the sauce will not set properly).
- When rested, add the olive oil a little at a time while turning (it would be nice to have someone to assist you). As you go, increase the flow of oil progressively while continuing to turn in the same direction.
- This sauce's consistency should be pretty thick. A teaspoon should stand up in it without falling.

✓ Chef's tip: I tried to use modern equipment for this recipe to avoid straining my wrist (hey, I'm not getting any younger, you know.) I did not have good success with a blender but it worked fairly well with an 8-10 oz food processor. Follow the same principles as above.

Sauce a l'Avocat. *Avocado Sauce*

This is kind of similar to guacamole, but French. I may hear grumbles form my Mexican friends, but I have had this in French restaurants. Did you know that, in French, avocat also means lawyer. Can we make a sauce out of lawyers? I wonder.

Servings: 4

Prep Time: 15 min.

INGREDIENTS

- **1 cup fresh tarragon leaves**
- **4 garlic cloves, peeled, degermed and chopped**
- **1 tsp sea salt**
- **½ tsp freshly ground white pepper**
- **4 ripe avocados**
- **4 Tbsp white wine vinegar**
- **1 cup extra virgin olive oil**

PROCEDURE

- Place the tarragon leaves, garlic and sea salt in the blender. Blend well, scraping down the sides of the bowl.

- Add the meat of the avocados. Blend until smooth.

- Through the top of the blender's lid, stream in the vinegar and finally the oil.

- Present in a nice bowl. Decorate with a few fresh tarragon leaves. Voila!

✓ Chef's tip: This sauce goes well with cold meats and white fish, as well as cold lobster or shrimp.

Sauce Citronnelle. *Lemon Cream Sauce*

This light sauce makes a great dipping sauce with fish. I like to use it as a vegetable dip as well.

Servings: 4

Prep Time: 10 min.

INGREDIENTS

- **The juice of two fresh lemons**
- **1 tsp Dijon mustard**
- **¼ tsp freshly ground white pepper**
- **½ tsp fine sea salt**
- **½ cup extra virgin olive oil**
- **4 Tbsp heavy whipping cream**

PROCEDURE

- Place the lemon juice, Dijon mustard, salt and pepper in a stainless steel, ceramic, or glass bowl. Whisk together.

- Add the olive oil progressively and create an emulsion by whisking energetically.

- Add the cream and continue to whisk briskly until the sauce is "fouettée" (whipped light).

✓ Chef's tip: You can accomplish similar results by using a blender, but you may have to double the recipe.

Desserts. *Desserts*

Pommes Cuites au Four avec Crème Chantilly. *Baked Apples with French Whipped Cream*

This is a warming dessert for the holidays, or any time you feel like a comforting dessert. The whipped cream adds a cloud of sweetness but can be omitted (I wouldn't!) C'est la touche finale (It's the final touch.)

Servings: 4

Prep Time: 10 min.

Cooking Time: 60 min.

INGREDIENTS

- **4 large organic apples, Granny Smith or Red Rome, halved and cored**
- **2 cups of your favorite granola**
- **2 Tbsp butter**

Whipped cream:

- **1/2 cup heavy whipping cream**
- **½ cup half-and-half**
- **1 oz raw sugar**
- **½ tsp vanilla extract**

PROCEDURE

- Preheat oven at 350°F.
- Place the halved and cored apples in a shallow baking dish (the apples should have a fairly large hole cut out of them in the center).
- Fill the holes in the apples with the granola mix (you may add seasonal fruits such as raisins, dried cranberries, nuts).
- Place a small dab of butter on top of the granola.
- Bake at 350 degrees for one hour.
- 5 minutes before the apples are done, whip the heavy cream, half and half, sugar and vanilla to soft peaks (you can also use heavy cream only).
- When apples are done, serve in individual bowls. Top each apple with a dollop of whipped cream.
- Serve while hot and before the whipped cream is completely melted. Yum!

✓ Chef's tip: The ½ heavy cream and ½ half-and-half will give you a lighter whipped cream called Crème Chantilly in French.

Souffle aux Framboises Léger comme un Nuage. *Light as a Cloud Raspberry Souffle*

This is a very healthy, very light, melt-in-the-mouth version of the traditional soufflé recipe. Unlike the traditional recipe, it does not contain any flour, just a touch of corn starch. I learned this recipe at a famous French health spa.

Servings: 4

Prep Time: 20 min.

Cooking Time: 12 min.

INGREDIENTS

- 4 - 3 3/4 " (7 3/4 fl oz) Le Creuset or other ceramic ramekins
- 4 oz raspberries fresh or frozen (about 1 cup)
- ¼ tsp fresh lemon juice
- ¼ cup powdered sugar
- ½ tsp corn starch

- 2 egg yolks
- 4 egg whites
- 1 pinch sea salt
- 2 Tbsp granulated sugar
- 2 Tbsp butter, at room temperature
- 2 Tbsp granulated sugar

PROCEDURE

- Preheat your oven at 400°F standard or 350°F convection.

- With a pastry brush, brush the inside of the ramekins with the softened butter. Sprinkle with granulated sugar. Turn the ramekins around to allow the sugar to stick evenly to the butter. Tap out the excess sugar gently.

- In a food processor or blender, blend the raspberries, sugar, cornstarch and lemon juice together. If you don't mind the seeds, leave this mix alone. Otherwise, strain the seeds out.

- Add the egg yolks to the fruit mixture. Blend well. Pour into a large mixing bowl.

- In a grease-free stand mixer bowl, start whisking the egg whites with the salt and sugar at medium speed, allowing them to fluff up gently. When all your ingredients are ready, increase the speed until they form soft peaks. Do NOT over whip, or they will form lumps while mixing.

- Add 1/3rd of the whipped egg whites into

Raspberry Sauce

- ½ **cup raspberries, fresh or frozen**
- ¼ **cup powdered sugar**
- ¼ **tsp fresh lemon juice**

the fruit mixture. Mix in gently with a hand whisk to lighten the mix. Add the rest of the egg whites and fold gently with a rubber spatula. With a spoon, carefully fill your prepared ramekins with the soufflé mixture. Level the tops carefully with a spatula or the back of a knife. With your right thumb, clean the inside edge of each ramekin to allow your soufflé to rise straight up.

- Bake at 400°F (350°F convection) for about 12 minutes or until the sides are light brown and firm to the touch.

- Sprinkle the top with powdered sugar and serve with the raspberry coulis or sauce (optional).

- **Raspberry Coulis**: process all ingredients in a food processor or blender. Strain through a fine mesh strainer or chinois. Refrigerate. Serve in a sauceboat with your hot soufflés. Pour sauce over soufflés just before eating. Bon Appétit!

✓ Chef's tips: You can replace the granulated sugar with finely processed turbinado sugar.
✓ The thin layer of butter spread inside the ramekins will allow the soufflé mixture to rise without sticking to the edge. The sprinkled sugar will bring an additional slight crunchiness to your soufflés. Be very careful not to allow your fingers to touch the inside of your ramekins once they have been prepared or your soufflé will stick and rise sideways.

Salade Rouge de Pamplemousse et Orange. *Red Grapefruit and Orange Salad*

This simple dessert is loaded with vitamin C, which is the one we need the most during Winter. A tasty way to ward off colds.

Servings: 4

Prep Time: 20 min.

INGREDIENTS

- **2 large pink grapefruits, peeled and quartered**
- **4 navel oranges, peeled and quartered**

- **Juice of 2 fresh oranges**
- **2 Tbsp local honey or raw agave nectar**
- **4 oz frozen raspberries (1/2 cup)**
- **The juice of 1 lemon**

PROCEDURE

- Peel the grapefruits and oranges with a small knife.

- Over a medium bowl, cut the citrus fruit into quarters, making sure to cut between the sections' skin. Squeeze out the juice remaining in the pulp. Drain the quarters, reserving the sections and the juice in separate bowls.

- In a food processor, place the drained juice, the juice of two additional oranges, the juice of one lemon, the honey and the frozen raspberries. Process together well. If you wish to avoid the raspberry seeds, strain the sauce over the quartered fruits. Toss lightly.

- Refrigerate for at least 30 minutes to allow the flavors to blend.

- Serve in bowls, topped with a fresh mint leaf.

✓ Chef's tip: This dessert is very refreshing after a heavy meal.

Salade de Fruits et sa Sauce au Gingembre. *Fruit Salad with Fresh Ginger Dressing*

This refreshing fruit salad is loaded with goodness: fiber, vitamin C and B. Add to that the exotic ginger flavor and your taste buds will want more!

Servings: 4

Prep Time: 20 min.

INGREDIENTS

Ginger sauce

- ½ cup fresh orange juice
- 1 Tbsp local honey or raw agave nectar
- 1 Tbsp fresh ginger, peeled and chopped fine

- 1 small pineapple, peeled, cored, and cubed (or buy it precut)
- 1 small cantaloupe, peeled and cubed
- 11 cups fresh strawberries
- 1 cup fresh blueberries

PROCEDURE

- Prepare the sauce first to allow your ingredients to macerate: mix the orange juice, honey and chopped ginger. Set aside.
- Slice off the top and bottom of your pineapple. Peel the outside skin with a serrated knife. Cut in quarters. Remove the core, and slice remaining pineapple in half-inch slices. Place in large mixing bowl.
- Cut your melon in half. Scoop out the seeds. Cut in eight sections. With a small knife, slice along the bottom of the melon, between the skin and the meat. Cut into half-inch chunks. Add to the mixing bowl.
- Rinse your strawberries in cold water and pat dry. Cut the green part off, and quarter. Add to bowl. Add the blueberries. Toss all the fruits together. Add the sauce and mix gently.
- Keep in your refrigerator for at least 30 minutes before serving to allow the flavors to blend.

Crêpes a l'Orange et au Grand Marnier. *Orange Grand Marnier French Crepes*

This recipe is always a winner at my yearly Mardi Gras crepe party. This is a modern version of a recipe Mamie taught me.

Servings: 4-6

Prep Time: 15 min.

Cooking Time: 30 min.

INGREDIENTS

- **2 ½ cups milk**
- **1 cup unbleached pastry flour**
- **4 Tbsp raw sugar**
- **4 eggs**
- **4 oz butter, melted (1 stick)**
- **The zest of one orange**
- **¼ cup Grand Marnier or Cointreau liquor**

PROCEDURE

– The reason I mentioned a modern version is because I prepare this recipe in my blender.

– Put the milk in the blender first. Add the flour, the sugar, orange zest, Grand Marnier and melted butter on top. Blend right away, first at low speed, then higher until it becomes smooth. If necessary, scrape the sides of the bowl with a rubber spatula.

– **Important**: Pour in a mixing bowl. Cover with a kitchen towel. Let rest for at least 30 minutes at room temperature to allow the flour to absorb the liquid and thicken.

– Heat an 8 or 9-inch frying pan, melt a little butter in it and spread thinly with a paper towel. Ladle 2 ounces of batter into your pan; rotate the batter quickly and evenly around the pan. Cook until the edges are turning light brown. With a metal spatula, pick up the crepe and flip carefully. If the batter is too thick, thin it down with water. Repeat until all the batter is used.

✓ Chef's tip: Everyone has their own favorite topping. My favorite is to sprinkle a little raw sugar and a little lemon juice and fold it. Miam!

Compote de Pruneaux au Vin Rouge et Cannelle. *Red Wine and Cinnamon Prune Compote*

I used to prepare this recipe as part of a compote cart at a few of the 4-star hotels where I used to work. Not only it is good for your digestive system, but it makes you slightly drunk. What's not to like?

Servings: 4

Prep Time: 10 min.

Cooking Time: 30 min.

INGREDIENTS

- **1 lb pitted prunes**
- **1 cup red wine**
- **1 cup filtered water**
- **8 oz local honey or raw agave nectar**
- **1 vanilla bean**
- **1 cinnamon stick**

PROCEDURE

- The day before, soak the prunes in the red wine and water in a saucepan. Cover with a kitchen towel and let sit overnight.

- The next day, add the honey or agave nectar, vanilla bean and cinnamon stick.

- Bring to boil, reduce the heat and let simmer for 30 minutes. Let cool to room temperature.

- Serve in glass coupes so you can see the prunes floating in the red wine. Enjoy and be regular.

✓ Chef's tip: If you feel like indulging, place two scoops of vanilla ice cream in a bowl. Add you prunes in wine, and yum, yum and triple-yum!

Tartes a la Crème au Citron a l'Anglaise et Meringue. *Tarts with English Lemon Curd and French Meringue*

I know, I know. This is an English recipe. I will not deny it. But I used to make these wonderful lemon curd tarts at Amandine French Bakery and my customers loved them. So in memory of my old bakery, here it is.

Servings: 4

Prep Time: 20 min.

Cooking Time: 20 min.

INGREDIENTS

- **6 egg yolks**
- **1 cup raw sugar**
- **Zest of 4 lemons**
- **Juice of 4 lemons (about ½ cup), strained**
- **4 oz unsalted butter, cold and cut in small pieces**

French meringue:

- **6 egg whites**
- **1 knife point of cream of tartar**
- **1 cup of granulated sugar**
- Whisk egg whites with cream of tartar until soft peaks form. Add sugar a little at a time while whisking until the meringue reaches firm peaks.

PROCEDURE

- Create a bain-marie (water bath) with a medium saucepan and a stainless steel bowl large enough to fit over the edge of the pan. Fill the saucepan with hot water to about one inch of the top of the pan. Bring to boil. Reduce heat to a gentle simmer.

- Wash and zest the lemons. Juice and strain to make a half-cup of juice. Juice more lemons if needed.

- In the stainless steel bowl, separate the yolks from the whites (save the whites for the French meringue). Whisk the yolks with the sugar until the mixture turns foamy and pale yellow. Whisk in the lemon juice and zest.

- Place the stainless steel bowl over the pot. Stir your custard constantly until the custard coats the back of your spatula. Do not boil or it will curdle.

- Take it away from the heat and add the cut butter one piece at a time while stirring to incorporate the butter. Cover with plastic film directly on the custard's surface so it will not get a skin. Refrigerate. Set oven to broil. Fill prebaked tart shells and top with French meringue. Broil to color the meringue.

Meringues au Cacao et aux Amandes. *Cocoa and Almond Meringues*

This dessert is light as air and perfect to go with your frozen desserts: ice cream or fruit sorbet. Or, if you can't wait for the sorbet, eat them as is. It contains a good amount of fiber from the nuts and antioxidants from the cocoa powder.

Servings: 4

20 meringues

Prep Time: 20 min.

Cooking Time: 20 min.

INGREDIENTS

- **2 egg whites**
- **A knife point of cream of tartar**
- **4 oz fine granulated sugar (about ½ cup)**
- **3 Tbsp unsweetened cocoa powder**
- **2 oz sliced almonds, (or chopped walnuts, pecan or hazelnuts), toasted**
- **2 baking pans fitted with parchment paper**
- **1 tablespoon or pastry bag fitted with a star tip.**

PROCEDURE

- Preheat your oven at 250°F.
- Prepare 2 baking sheet pans with parchment paper.
- On a separate sheet pan, toast your almonds until golden-colored.
- The best way to prepare this recipe is with a stand mixer, if you have one.
- This meringue is called a French meringue (it's true, I promise! If you want to know more, visit one of my classes).
- Place your egg whites and cream of tartar in the mixing bowl. Start mixing on medium speed while you prepare the rest of your ingredients. Weigh the sugar in a measuring cup.
- Sift the cocoa powder into a bowl. Add your toasted almonds. Mix together.
- When everything is ready, increase the speed of your mixer to high. As soon as it looks light and fluffy, add your sugar progressively until it forms firm peaks. Fold in the cocoa powder and almonds.
- Drop dollops of meringue on your baking pans. Separate them to allow for expansion. Bake for 1 hour, door ajar, at 250°F until dry. Cool and store in a box with a tight lid.

Gâteau au Fromage et à la Citrouille. *Pumpkin Cheese Cake*

I once brought this cheesecake to my church for the Thanksgiving brunch. They've been raving about it ever since and request it every year. Of course, it is prideful of me to be happy about this, but who said I was a saint?

Servings: 8

Cake size: 9 inch

Prep Time: 20 min.

Cooking Time: 2 ½ hours

INGREDIENTS

Crust:

- 10 oz graham crackers
- 4 oz (1 stick) butter, melted

Cheese cake filling:

- 1.5 lbs Organic Valley cream cheese
- 12 oz Organic Valley sour cream
  ½ cup raw sugar
- 2 Tbsp cornstarch
- 2 tsp ground cinnamon
- 1.5 tsp ground ginger
- ½ tsp ground nutmeg
- 1 lb 4 oz Organic canned pumpkin puree
- 4 whole eggs, beaten

PROCEDURE

- Preheat your oven at 250°F.

- Wrap a piece of aluminum foil around the outside of the bottom and sides of the spring-form pan.

- Grind the graham cookies with the melted butter in a food processor fitted with a metal blade.

- Press into the bottom of the spring-form pan. Bake at 250°F for 8 minutes; turn around, bake for another 8 minutes. Allow to cool.

- Whisk sugar, cornstarch and spices together.

- Wash the food processor's bowl. Fit with metal blade again. Add cream cheese. Cream with the sugar, cornstarch and spice mix until smooth.

- Blend in the sour cream.

- Add pumpkin puree. Blend in.

- Add sea salt and vanilla to the eggs. Whisk together.

- Add eggs/salt/vanilla to cheesecake;

- ¼ **tsp sea salt**
- **2 tsp vanilla extract**

mix a little at a time at low speed

- Pour mix into the pan. Place the cake pan in an oven dish. Pour hot water around cake pan. Place in oven.

- Bake at 250°F for 1.5 hour – turn around – then 1 hour at 200°F. Let cool overnight. Turn out of the pan and serve cold.

Sorbet aux Pèches de Fredericksburg. *Fredericksburg Peach Sorbet*

I love this recipe for a refreshing dessert during the hot Texas summer. I offer you two versions: the traditional sorbet and the quick sorbet. Feel free to substitute your favorite local brand of peaches in season. Enjoy!

Servings: 6

Prep Time: 20 min.

Cooking Time: 20 min.

INGREDIENTS

Agave syrup:

- **1 pint hot water**
- **12 oz pure raw agave nectar**

- **3 lbs ripe peaches, local if possible (Fredericksburg peaches are the best around Austin)**
- **1 lemon juice per pound of peach slices**
- **1 egg white per batch**

- **Pre-frozen ice cream dishes or coupes**

PROCEDURE

- In a small pot, stir agave nectar into the hot water. Bring to boil. Cool down. Use cold.
- Use ripe peaches for better flavor.
- To peel, plunge the peaches into boiling water until their skins loosen. Then drop them into iced water. Drain and peel. Cut into halves, take the pits out and slice thin.
- In a food processor's bowl, weigh 1 pound of peach slices; add 8 oz of agave syrup and the juice of one lemon.
- Process all ingredients until pureed. Strain the puree through a chinois or fine sieve.
- Cool the puree in your refrigerator for at least one hour before freezing.
- Freeze in an ice cream machine or sorbetière according to the manufacturer's instructions. It should take about 20 minutes.
- If you want your sorbet to be smoother, towards the end of the freezing process, add a beaten egg white to the sorbet machine and finish freezing.
- Scoop into the pre-frozen ice cream dishes.
- Decorate artistically with a few fresh

- **Mint leaves for decoration**
- **Fresh raspberries for decoration**

- **Optional: Peach brandy or champagne**

raspberries and mint leaves.

Optional: If you feel festive, pour a small amount of cold peach brandy or champagne over the scooped sorbet and decorate.

QUICK PEACH SORBET

Although this makes a decent substitute sorbet, it will not be as smooth and light as the original version. It'll be more like a thick smoothie. Enjoy!

- Buy already frozen organic peach slices.
- Prepare your agave syrup as above.
- Weigh the frozen peaches, syrup and egg white in the same proportions as above, and process together quickly.
- Put back in the freezer for at least one hour before scooping out.
- Serve and decorate as above.

ACKNOWLEDGMENTS

This book represents both my love for food and my interest in nutrition. I would like to thank all of the following special people for their inspiration and support through all phases of this project. My very special thanks to:

My grand-mother **"Mamie"** for teaching me by example that healthy food should come from one's kitchen garden, freshly picked, prepared quickly but with love but does not have to be complicated to taste wonderful.

My mother, **Bernadette Moulin-Braux,** who encouraged me to discover and apply my culinary and baking abilities. My mother-in-law, **Helene Jaboulay,** for opening my eyes to what Mediterranean cuisine is all about. She always amazed me with her ability to feed her family with simple but flavorful home-cooked "cuisine du Sud".

The dear **Janet Zand** for being my first supporter even before I started writing the first word. I went to her to present the idea of this book and she enthusiastically encouraged me to put pen to paper. Throughout this project, she was my mentor, my inspiration and my muse. Thank you Janet.

My very creative team: **Kathleen Thornberry** for her loving editing. When it comes to food and arts, we are kindred spirits and this project would have been almost impossible without her astute suggestions and reinterpretation of my "Frenchisms" while preserving the spirit of my writing. **Athena Danoy** for capturing that special spark in me in her portraits and offering her vision for the book's cover. **Nathan Stueve** for designing a beautiful and practical web site and an original book cover. Their creative efforts supported my vision for this book. I literally could not have done without them.

My esteemed predecessors and guiding mentors: **Hippocrates** 460-377 B.C., the father of us all in the "food as a healing medium" movement, who affirmed, "Let thy food be thy medicine and thy medicine be thy food"; **Dr. Joanna Budwig**. 1908-2003., the first modern scientist to discover the connection between damaging industrial oils and human health; **Dr. Catherine Kousmine,** for measuring the effects of industrial food on mice and proving that "modern" food is dangerous for us; **Dr. Seignalet,** 1936-2003, for his lifelong commitment to treating his clients with his ancient diet, and proving that food can actually heal degenerative diseases. And finally my daily inspiration for writing this book: **Jonny Bowden, Ph. D.** and **George Mateljan**. My Chef's hat off to both of you for proving that we can still hack it even if we're not in our 20's.

Bill Swail for providing me the safety and security I needed during the writing of this book. Also for supporting this endeavor with his astute marketing advice.

Kimberly Freeman for sharing her amazing online promotion savvy with me. **Valerie Hausladen** for believing that my dream to teach health through food was a good dream, despite my doubts. **Julia Bower** for being my constant cheerleader, "maman poule" and ciné buddy. **Kim Stanford** for her enthusiastic support through this project.

Tim and Barbara Cook for their spiritual guidance and encouragements.

Thank you **Brigitte Benquet** and **Ivan Semeniuk** for opening your house, offering props and your love for food to help us create the front cover.

To my kitty girl, **Piou Piou**, for 20 years of faithful companionship. I just wish you'd learn how to clean up after yourself. Oh well! You can't have it all.

Almost last but by no means least, my son **Gilles Braux** for inspiring me to be the best I can, just by being and staying himself no matter what. We've been through a lot together and I am proud of the loving relationship we have been able to develop. I am proud of your accomplishments too, "my favorite son in the whole wide world".

And finally, my **Foodie Fans** and **Cholesterol Champions** that have been supporting me through my belief that fresh and good-tasting food is the source of good health. Thanks for all you're doing.

Love and Dark Chocolate. Chef Alain Braux.